Spa-Cipes
The Spa Cookbook

Written by

Melissa Stone Santangelo

Spa-Cipes
Copyright April 1, 2014

ISBN-13: 978-1494253073 &
ISBN-10: 1494253070

Printed in the United States of America

Requests for information should be addressed to:
Melissa Stone Santangelo
at
melissa@balancestudio.org
Cover design work, interior design work and editing
by Daniel Gross

Dragonfly Publishing Company
Felton, CA

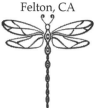

None of the statements in this book have been evaluated by the FDA.
None of the statements in this book should be construed as dispensing
medical advice or making claims regarding the cure of diseases. You
should consult a licensed health care professional before starting any
cleanse, or diet/exercise program, especially if you are pregnant or have
any pre-existing injuries or medical conditions.

Professional Reviews for Spa-Cipes

Melissa Stone Santangelo's Spa-Cipes is an engaging and informative book for everyone who wants to feel good, look good and be environmentally conscious at the same time.

Melissa brings her knowledge of herbs and foods into a warm and informative approach to caring for yourself and/or your loved one in the comfort of your own home. She does a great job of explaining the ingredients and why each one is beneficial. The recipes are easy and exciting to prepare and use.

Melissa delights in offering the wisdom she has discovered about our bodies, minds, herbs and foods in ways that are fun and helpful. This is a book infused with Love for all and makes taking care of yourself easier than you might think.
Try a few of the recipes-you'll be glad you did!

Larry Bernstein
Cypress Health Institute

I have known Melissa for some years, so I already knew she was on the path of enlightenment and balance. She asked me to preview her wonderful new book, and I must say I have seldom read something so profoundly simple, yet powerful.

All in one book, she has designed a way to live that offers a very understandable way to live holistically. Frankly, it was so exciting that I had to reread it to grasp the elegant simplicity of it; she has taken a very complex process, and reduced it to something we can start using immediately. This book will change your life. It is as beautifully present, as simply complex and balanced as Melissa herself.
To get something you never had ...Do something you've never done".

Theo Jackson
Family Therapist

Spa-Cipes is an insightful and fun way to treat yourself to a spa treatment and increase your own well-being. Melissa is an amazing Creatrix of culinary spa recipes and techniques. She has learned how to balance and pamper the soul to perfection. It is such a beautiful gift and blessing that she shares all of her life long experience and expertise in Spa-Cipes. Taking ingredients from the Kitchen not only makes spa luxuries affordable and accessible to all, it keeps it natural and chemical free. Blending in meditation, Melissa gets to every need of our soul for rejuvenation and relaxation. Spa-Cipes helps you create a space and mindset that will make you rejuvenated and exhilarated.

Inara Sophia
CMT, Reiki Master/Teacher, Holistic Practitioner

In Spa-Cipes, Melissa combines multiple aspects of living life in balance with simple and easy to follow in-home recipes for a variety of skin, body and emotional well being. She covers a multitude of holistic bath, body and meditation techniques for life's every day physical and emotional challenges. It is apparent her life's journey has been instrumental in the development of these recipes and techniques to become an accomplished spa solutions expert. In addition to approaching emotional and physical well being from the outside using natural food sources, healing salts and oils, she completes the circle with nutritional and dietary solutions. I was very impressed with the overall scope and depth of this book. An excellent home health reference as well as a wonderful gift for friends and family.

Mary Vernier
Mary's Green and Clean Handcrafted Soaps

I love all things related to plants and the natural world. Being a landscape designer and gardening columnist I am always outside with flowers, trees and fragrance. When I read Melissa's book I was happy to see how she had woven their uses into our daily life. Her Spa-Cipes and recipe for happiness in life is infectious.

There is a saying in the Lakota tribe that reads "When a man moves away from nature his heart becomes hard." Melissa's book not only gives you a recipe for living and enjoying a healthy life, she has peppered it with inspirational sayings that brighten your day. One of my favorites is by Charles Schultz and reads: "All you need is love. But a little chocolate now and then doesn't hurt."

Melissa's book contains recipes for scented baths that relax or energize you, foot soaks, shower soothers, room sprays, homemade soaps, food facials, hair treatments, detox wraps, healing body treatments for us and our pets as well as shopping lists for natural foods and an explanation for how they help our bodies. There are also recipes for healthful smoothies, snacks and meals.

I loved Spa-Cipes and recommend it to everyone who enjoys nature as I do. And who doesn't love to surround themselves with flowers, fruit, and healthy vegetables in new and creative ways?

Jan Nelson
The Mountain Gardener
and gardening columnist for The Press Banner

After reading Spa-Cipes, all I can say is... *FINALLY*! Set-N-Me-Free has encouraged the innovative use of natural food ingredients to improve skin in a safe and effective way, for over thirty years. Melissa has made this concept a reality with her new book. This beautiful collection of recipes and techniques are *simple* enough for the home spa and *effective* enough for the professional to use on clients in the fanciest spa.

Nicol Sockey
Set-N-Me-Free Aloe Vera

CONTENTS

Dedication

Hailey Stone, Dress up and spa time were fun times!

Barbarajean Santangelo, just like a Mother to shape a daughters life.

With all my Love to Daniel Gross, it's about time you showed up!

A Special Thank You
To Michael Steinrok for giving me the Spa-Cipes name.

Forward

There's little question that science and technology have contributed greatly to improving life here on planet Earth. Medical advances such as the artificial heart, prolongs the lives of those that might otherwise die while waiting for a transplant. More than 20,000,000 people have watched the YouTube video of Sarah Churman's wonderment at hearing for the first time, thanks to a cochlear implant. The Internet has made it possible for people to connect with one another to share, work, learn and rally together as if they lived in the same town and not halfway around the world. Yet there is a dark side to modern progress.

Today's Standard American Diet (SAD) is comprised of processed, fatty, sugar-laden and dead foods that contribute to chronic illnesses such as diabetes, heart disease and obesity. Corporate giants manufacture foodstuffs loaded with genetically-modified organisms and artificial ingredients, which are toxic to people and animals. Products on labels of personal care products found in the neighborhood drug store require a PhD in science to decipher, having been invented in a test tube. Even the terms "earth-friendly" and "'natural" have been bastardized by large corporations to green wash products that are anything but earth-friendly and natural.

The good news is that we are, in my opinion, enjoying a renaissance - a return to what is truly healthy, simple and sustainable. More and more people in the mainstream are waking up not only to the dangers of our modern world, but also to alternative lifestyles and products that were the norm for our grandparents and great-grandparents. One of the gifts of the Internet is that information can be shared not solely by those with the deepest pockets and greatest political power, but by the meekest among us, at a grass roots level. In the end, knowledge is power. People are growing their own food, even in urban areas where wide open spaces are non-existent. New Meetup groups focusing on spiritual, financial and physical fitness are formed every day, providing opportunities for exercise, community and improvement in these areas. And, they're available to anyone with access to a computer with Internet access, including those at public libraries.

Spa-Cipes is a true example of not only what is truly healthy but also of the natural health and beauty renaissance happening today. The recipes in this book make it incredibly easy not only for people to take better care of themselves and their families, but to do so . Users of these spa-cipes will not only benefit from the healing power of the ingredients, but they will also be contributing to lessening their impact on the environment – and having fun in the process!

It is both inspiring and admirable when an individual like Melissa Stone Santangelo is able to connect so easily and deeply with her childhood-self. As a child, she found herself in the kitchen mixing up batches of spa treatments using food from her pantry and refrigerator.

Melissa was divinely connected to the contents of her mother's kitchen! She concocted and tested and revised her creations until they were the best they could be. Melissa has been using these recipes at her spa for many years, much to the delight of her clients. Now, Melissa is graciously sharing the best of these proven formulas with her clients and fans. For that, Melissa gets a gold star in my book!

Janet Lancaster
Earth's Living Clay
San Diego, California

Introduction

This book is a great place to find holistic recipes to cleanse the body inside and out. I have been asked many times, what do I put in my food facial?" and "what foods are best to use on my face?" Hearing these questions every day prompted me to put all my Spa-Cipes down on paper.

    I use these recipes in my everyday life and my spa practice. After you try one or two recipes, add in your own favorite foods and herbs. If you don't like something I have in a recipe, just take it out. The beauty of "spa- ing" in your kitchen is that there are no rules, only suggestions from what has worked in my experience. With this book, I hope to light a passion within you for taking care of yourself. My first book, The Key To Life Is Balance was a way for me to put my healing journey down on paper and to share what I've learned to help heal any heaviness in your heart. Spa-Cipes is my second book and it's one people can really have fun with or to heal many wounds, much like I did as a kid.

    With The Key To Life Is Balance, journaling my thoughts was a great way for me to really find out what I needed to work on to heal myself. My own journaling, the tools I used, and the stories in it helped me shape my healing practice, but more importantly, my life. I want to help everyone by giving out the knowledge I've learned. In my books, you'll find easy tips that can help you enjoy life to the fullest, in the present moment.

Believe first that you are worth taking care of and that you have time to give to yourself. Use everything that works for you and throw out what does not fit. Learning from other people's healing experiences are a wonderful way to explore what can work for you, too. Find out how they came to reach their goals, and then emulate their success. Knowledge is power!

Recently, I was listening to Wayne Dyer speak and he said, "You have to start with willingness to make any changes in your life." He is correct. Any time I am willing to do something, I complete it. I get to the finish line every time and in my life I feel I have accomplished a lot of good with my willingness. Not just for me but higher good, for everyone. Anyone that wants to learn to be better to themselves and looks within for that change to occur will make change in a higher vibrational way. I feel very Blessed about my openness to being willing. I know you are willing to spa because you took that first step and bought the book which you are now reading. Congratulations for being willing to give these treatments and love to yourself! I feel honored that you would be willing to make my recipes in your home. This brings me great Joy and keeps me writing. I love teaching self care to everyone I meet!

This is what I was meant to do, I feel it deep within me. I knew it as a child, but forgot as a teen and young adult.

I decided to write this spa cookbook as a gift to you, giving you the insights to what you, too, can do to help your skin, hair and body look and feel its best. Now is the time on my path of healing for sharing. Sharing my knowledge in one place for you to enjoy! Have fun and invite over some friends, make a food facial and spa right in your kitchen! Or make them when you have a heavy heart and see how easy it is to heal yourself. You will find out a lot about what really works for you by playing with all the recipes when feeling good and when you are feeling not so good.

Mix them together and add your own flare. Enjoy this journey of discovering what food looks good on your hair, face and body and what cleanses the inside as well. Food is the resource Mother Nature has put in place for us to be nourished to live a healthy life. Herbs are grown for the enhancement of the taste of foods but can be also be used as medicinal teas. Both food and herbs are what heal us and keep us healthy, and give our body what it needs to live.

Food and herbs also serve a purpose in our beauty as well. I believe what naturally grows on Earth is our medicine and can be used to heal skin, hair and keep us beautiful. Plants have been placed here for our survival and growing older and aging can seem like a survival mission, too!

When we ingest the things that grow on Earth that keep us in balance, it keeps us healthy on the inside. This helps us to survive and thrive. But, what about the outside? Are you placing harmful chemicals on to your skin? Did you know that some skin care products can cause PMS and imbalances in hormones? That got me thinking twice about what I was really putting on my skin. I have been doing food facials for a long time, but I also have been using store bought products for years. I dye my hair every six weeks and I was using store bought shampoos, conditioners and face products. Do they give me the results they claim? Maybe, but also what harm are these chemicals doing to my body chemistry?

If you think about early times, there were no stores, no restaurants, and you couldn't just buy your skin care products. Instead, there were farmers and farmer's wives that made soap and would use salt to heal a tired farmer's body by adding it to his bath. I can see it coming full circle. Clients, neighbors and friends tell me they are growing food to save money and to feed healthy organic food to their families.

Canning is also becoming very popular again. This year. we made mustard for Christmas gifts. I was so surprised at how easy it is and everyone loved it! Have we let companies tell us we are too busy to make our own products?

I am making about 90% of my skin care products and it is easy. Since I am using food for my skin care and for my clients treatments, sometimes I find myself making a facial mask and my lunch all at the same time. I'll be making breakfast and see my face needs some toning and tightening, so I'll set aside part of the egg. I am excited to be placing these Spa-Cipes all here in an organized way for anyone to start using them right away.

You can heal your skin and body from the chemicals and skin care products that are creating imbalances in your body. After reading an article about the chemicals in skin care products a few years ago, I started to think about what I was putting on my skin and how my body was continually having some hormonal imbalances. I was suffering from adult acne and horrible PMS. "Maybe it's the skin care products," I thought. I was using a lot of them and nothing was working; every month mood swings, horrible breakouts and painful cramps. I have healed all of these by not using any of the skin care products anymore on my face and by using clay, food and herbs. My hair is thicker and shinier than ever before because I use food and oils, not hair care products. The best part is that I'm saving my hard earned money. I already buy the food I am using on my skin and hair to eat. I will one day grow these foods and herbs and then that will save me more money. Best of all, I will know that what I am ingesting and placing on my skin is clean of any chemicals and made with Love.

Throughout this book, I will be guiding you on how you can pamper yourself from things in your own garden and kitchen. I hope you can get to a place of doing at home spa treatments each night, along with drinking smoothies for at least one meal. If you decide to do the Balance 7 Day Juice Cleanse in Chapter Nine, think about adding in a spa treatment each day as well. You will feel a difference if you commit at least 15 (preferably 30) minutes every morning and every night to do some guided meditation, facials, body & foot wraps, detox baths and salt scrubs right out of your garden and kitchen. This is living! You will start to look and feel amazing! This is what I call taking care of yourself, in the highest vibrational way. When you are taking care of yourself, you are taking care of the world. We are One! Everything in our world is an extension of us. If you want to take care of others, you MUST first take care of yourself. Remember what they tell you on an airplane, "In an emergency, place the mask on yourself first, then help others. " Well I say, "Take care of yourself first! Then help others!"

Chapter One
Spa Memories

I can remember a time when I hated myself, and all the thoughts that ran through my head were all about how unworthy I was to have anything. This feels like a lifetime ago and to my delight I was able to get past these thoughts without therapy, medications or falling down in too deep of a hole. I am very proud of my remarkable recovery, from loathing my body to loving it! How did I do that? I did it through meditation and sometimes meditation with a food facial!

I love to spa and my spa-ing abilities came out at a very early age. My Mom loves reading the weekly tabloids that they sell at the check stands. In the living room by her chair, there were lots of Woman's Day, The Enquirer, Women's World and these types of magazines. There are lots of spa recipes in them, and when I was bored and not happy with myself I would test them out. I spent many years doing this and, let me tell you, I learned that food not only nourishes you on the inside, it heals you on the outside! A food mask spread out on the face will disappear before your eyes as the skin soaks it in fast. Skin recognizes this is good for it and it clearly is the most effective natural way to keep your skin healthy! But the biggest side effect was that I felt happy with myself after a spa treatment, even if it was at home. This quickly became my happy place when I was down and it still is to this day.

I spent a lot of years not understanding why my life felt absent of love. Using spa treatments helped me to learn how to love myself. It also taught me that I could fix myself, and that I did not need to shop, drink, or use drugs or sex to make myself happy. I found my real authentic self while spa-ing. I have cried with facials on, I have used them as celebration and I always use them to get ready for a date out on the town. I know my self-loathing and feeling lost was all to make ME who I am today! It all dawned on me when I was on my healing journey. Letting go of all of that grief and abandonment did help me to get back into balance. The spa treatments were a way to spend time with myself and I know you could use time with yourself. This is why I wrote this book, to give you a big huge excuse to spa in your kitchen and learn to love yourself.

I would not change my path for the world, but there was a time that I made up stories and played pretend. I used to mix lotions, bath products and pretend I was selling products and giving advice on how to help yourself look and feel great. Now that I think back, everything I did as a kid, I am doing now as my career. Funny how that happens.

"Never Let Your Memories Be Bigger
Than Your Dreams"

- Doug Ivestor

When I was seven, I remember slathering Noxzema all over my body while explaining it as a treatment to myself. It was before school and I remember feeling odd and not wanting to go. It felt like I was late for school and I was doing my treatment for a long time before my Mom came in the room. There I was, naked with Noxzema spread all over my body. My Mom was mad, yelling at me, "What have you DONE?", washing me off and getting me dressed all at the same time.

Years later, I remember making up facial masks out of oatmeal and clay and I would wash my hair in mayonnaise. At a young age, I knew to look in the kitchen for treatments to make my loneliness and pain fall away.

I was always in trouble by my Mother or some neighborhood mom because of mixing together the bathroom and kitchen products into potions. This obsession to mix and apply to my skin was not something anyone nurtured at all. One Christmas, the adults were in the kitchen, and my brother, a cousin and myself were in the back of the house. I was about 8 and I was admiring these bath beads that I knew had oil in them. I started to squish one in my fingers and it popped. I popped a few more and then tried to rub it on my brother and my cousin, chasing them around with this oil all over my hands. My Aunt came in the room, and boy, was I in trouble!

Being in trouble never deterred me from my passion about spa treatments. In 1996, I found myself getting a divorce and becoming a single Mother with a two year old. Your self esteem really drops when you are in this situation, even when it is amicable. I started a ritual of Friday nights being *my* night instead of date night. I would give spa time to myself, and then I would look beautiful when I met a guy to go on a date with. It was my thought process to keep myself looking good and do something good for me instead of feeling sorry for myself. I would first pluck my eye brows, do my nails, fingers, and toes, and soak my feet. Then, to top it all off, a facial and hot bath. By the time I was done, Friday night was over, and I could go to sleep feeling good. At times, my daughter would want her nails done and then we would play dress up and laugh.

I have kept the dream alive and I am still creating potions of healing from food and herbs. In 2003, I created my dream job at Balance Studio Spa, where I still offer my signature food facials and body treatments to clients from all over Northern California. I created a job that I could do at home so I could be raising my pre-teen daughter and do what I love all at the same time.

I feel I am sort of a Kitchen Witch, always learning about different ways to treat problem skin and increase my own well-being using pastes, masks and baths. These remedies will deliver what you ask of them and they will comfort your every relaxing, renewing, and refreshing need. I have given myself many facials, healing many rashes, bug bites and acne over the years. I have seen thousands of people in my spa setting and have helped in the healing of these clients using food and herbs, all from my kitchen. There is one thing that all my spa clients have in common. They were all in need of some unconditional love and I truly believe my treatments gave that to them.

We deplete ourselves everyday by giving too much, over-extending our energy to make others happy. Do you take time to rejuvenate? Most people do not and the feeling may become so overwhelming that mood swings, illness, or pain in the body can begin. These are all sign of being depleted. These signs tell us we need some attention, some relaxation and love. We actually want it and need it from ourselves. This is when you may misread the signs and distract yourself with shopping or trying to find someone to love you. What is really needed is some time to yourself.

Give a little bit of spa time to yourself each and every day. It will become a routine that you automatically go to. After some time of having spa time with yourself, you will want to look a bit deeper. It won't be so hard to take a look when you are emerged in a hot lavender bath and have a chocolate avocado mask on. You will want to meet and get to know this person you are spending spa time with.

My earliest memory of looking within was about the age of five when I had no one else to turn to. It was not until my 40's when I found what I call my *Groovy Goddess*. She is the part of me that is authentic and real. She knows no shyness and self loathing. She is confident with everything she does. She is sexy and fun. Having high integrity, she is loyal and trusts the Universe completely. She is complete LOVE!

I do love to analyze myself, my behaviors and to look at why I do things. I love the subject of self help, as I had to seek it all my life. When you have to seek out to get answers because there is no one giving you any, the answers will show up for you. Be open to looking!

You can become an expert in yourself when you incorporate the answers you find and not just stuffing it all back down again. I love to help others find their own Groovy Goddess, like I found mine! This book is my way to help all the ladies (and men!) in the world drop the draining way of living and start to discover the inner Goddess or God that lies within them!

One way to finding your inner Goddess or God is to SPA! And, it's the most fun way of all! You can do therapy if you want and keep talking about your stuff over and over again or you can spa it all away. I do suggest using spa time to be alone with yourself for some time. You can spa with girlfriends later on when you have found yourself a bit. But for now, keep it your own special thing and use it to stop the negative talk.

Think about it, you look in the mirror and see a
blemish and all of a sudden the negative thoughts start
to flow in. You are ugly, fat and do not deserve
anything good. Some of us start our days like this. I
remember doing it myself for years.

The way I like to start my day is in the present,
by looking in the mirror. If I see a blemish, I know that I
have the power to mix something together to fix it all
by myself. I don't have the negative talks with myself
like I used to in the past. It is more about finding what
I need and then using it to heal.

When you start to spa, you don't need to get this
deep with yourself at all! You can simply think "I need
some *me* time", find a spa recipe that resonates with
what you are feeling in this moment, and enjoy!
Just remember, spa time is always there to help you to
change things about yourself that you really want to
change. All you have to do is get relaxed in your spa
mask, bathe with scented candles and start asking
questions of yourself. If you listen and stay relaxed
enough without judging what you hear, you will learn
a lot.

When you are giving yourself spa treatments
daily, you show the shy little girl or boy inside that you
love her or him. The love is coming from where you
really want it to come from, yourself, and you relax,
and in that place you heal. When you heal, you will
begin to love yourself, really Love yourself. It is quite
amazing!

When you truly love yourself, you will start saying yes to the things in life that nourish and nurture you. You will easily speak your truth, learn from your mistakes, and most of all, you will start to take really good care of yourself.

As I write this book, I am at the age where my Mom is a senior and we are going through her health issues. I feel like my Mom does not take loving care of herself. She will stuff emotional issues down and worries about a lot of things that are out of her control. My Mom shapes my life because I see her struggles. I adjust my thinking and openness to do things that keep me away from these struggles.

There comes a time when all of the things you stuff down come up and you explode with anger or sadness, and health issues can arise. After care-giving for my Mom when she broke her hip in 2011, I started to think about my own health.

I wanted to do a full body cleanse at the time, but needed to have energy to do my job and be a caregiver for my Mom. I could not be drained and feeling sick while detoxing and cleansing my body. I searched for a cleanse that would be effective and still let me do what I needed to do during the day.

This is how I created the Balance 7 Day Juice Cleanse. Having interviewed Jack LaLanne on my radio show back in 2008, I remembered asking him what he ate. I started to think about most of his philosophies and how he kept himself healthy and strong. He told me his secrets during that radio show (I have this archived on my web site at http://www.balancestudio.org/media.php), and I used what he told me as a basis for the cleanse you will read in Chapter Nine. I started to look at the issues that were going on in my body at the time, like congestion, inflammation and pain from over use of muscles. At the top of the list was the feeling of being rundown and tired.

I know that this low energy and all the other symptoms I was having were just an over load of toxins. Sugar, gluten and milk were also found to be culprits in my sluggishness and inflammation.

After a year of following the cleanse I created, I look and feel great, and more committed than ever to staying on track with my eating habits, exercise and taking care of myself. I hope this book helps you reach a blissful state of reflection, relaxation, and healing!

Here's to your HEALTH!
Enjoy these recipes and build many lovely spa memories!

- Melissa

Chapter Two
Soothing Soaks and Healing Baths

One of life's simple pleasures is a hot bath! A long hot soak in the tub can do wonders for your body and your frame of mind. A simple bath will reduce stress and anxiety as soon as your toe hits the hot water. Taking a soothing soak is the easiest solution to many issues of muscle pain and body fatigue, too.

Healing baths can also be a foot bath, simply make a smaller version of the soothing soak recipe to create a nice relaxing foot bath. Reflexology is a type of foot massage. Based on what reflexologists claim, our feet are a system of zones and reflex areas that reflect an image of the body on the feet, with the premise that such work effects a physical change to the body. Just by rubbing your feet you can help relieve pain and fatigue all over your body. Next time you find yourself without a bath tub, just place your feet into hot water with the relaxing herbs and let the foot bath give your whole body a relaxing feeling.

I like to create a healing bath of herbs, salt and oils that will help with what I am feeling at the time. These recipes will give you many choices to create the soaks that help you with stress, muscle ache, colds and much more.

Have your soaking room ready to go so that when you want to take your healing bath you will not let excuses like "It's a lot of work" or "I don't have all the stuff" keep you from having your bath. I promise you that taking the time now to clean your bathroom, get it organized and fully stocked with all you need for healing baths will make it easier for you to do this for yourself.

Placing ambient light around your tub with your candles just makes it more special. You can use candles that have relaxing scents like lavender or vanilla to give your room the scent of freshness.

Find what you and your family like and then keep them close by. If you don't like to have many candles around for fire reasons, you can get the LED battery operated candles. These are nice as some of them have a timer and you can set your lighting to turn on as you run your water each night. I use my LED timer candles as a night light because they go on the same time each night and stay on for five hours. This way, my bathroom is always lit up in the middle of the night when I need to get up and I am half asleep.

After you have your lighting set up in your soaking room, you can work on setting up your soaking supplies. Having your placement of candles, oils and herbs near your tub will make bath time a easy pleasure. Set up a cabinet or drawer with your essential oils, salts and bubble baths.

Have a wide variety in your supply at all times. Look over the following recipes and find which ones you will want to do most often. Always remember when choosing your essential oils that you are using oils that are skin safe. Some oils are for burning and are not safe to use on your skin. Be aware of the products you are using by making sure the ingredients in them are safe for your skin.

When choosing your oils, research what scents help what problems. For instance, lavender will relax you and eucalyptus helps with congestion and cough.

Essential oils are derived from sections of plants. Some plants, like the bitter orange, are sources of several types of essential oil. I am adding a list here for you to follow easily. Have some of your favorites on hand and ready for use in your soaking room.

List of essential oils

Berries
Allspice and Juniper

Seeds
Almond, Anise, Buchu, Celery, Cumin, Nutmeg oil, Bark, Cassia, Cinnamon and Sassafras

Wood
Camphor, Cedar, Rosewood, Sandalwood and Agarwood

Rhizome
Ginger

Leaves
Basil, Bay leaf, Buchu, Cinnamon,Common sage,
Eucalyptus, Guava, Lemon grass, Melaleuca, Oregano
Patchouli, Peppermint, Pine, Rosemary, Spearmint,
Tea tree, Thyme, Tsuga and Wintergreen

Resin
Benzoin, Copaiba, Frankincense, Myrrh Flowers,
Cannabis, Clary sage, Chamomile, Clove, Scented
geranium, Hops, Hyssop, Jasmine, Lavender, Manuka
Marjoram, Orange, Rose and Ylang-ylang

Peel
Bergamot, Grapefruit, Lemon, Lime, Orange and
Tangerine

Root
Valerian

I'd like to give you some insight on a few oils that I use often and why. If you are curious about the other oils, just do a Google search and you can get that information.

Rose is a great scent to use when you have a heavy heart. Rose has the highest vibration to its scent and this scent alone will help to heal your Heart Chakra. Helping you through the tough times, this scent brings me back to my childhood and comforts me. We had a bottle of Rose Milk lotion next to the sink when I was a kid.

When I smell this scent now, it gives me a sweet, comforting feeling. I use a spray of Rose when my heart is heavy and it uplifts me quickly. I do like to inspire people to use scents to help uplift the moods and comfort. A hot soak with rose, adding in a rose salt scrub will help give you the feeling of being loved. I have healed my own many broken hearts myself using the scent of rose. I will go into more of my favorite scents in Chapter Six when we will play with salt scrubs.

Being Grounded is something we all need to be a bit more aware of. I will go into this more later in this chapter. Sandalwood is a nice scent for this and Sage is my favorite for cleansing away negativity.

I also like to have fresh flowers in my bathroom at all times and several sprays that can fill the room with wonderful scents to smell while I fill my tub. We will go into room sprays and how to make them later in this Chapter.

The last item you should have to complete your soaking space is some soaps that you like. I am not a soap maker, so I asked a local soap maker **Mary Vernier** for her soap recipes. She was wonderful and listed out several soap processes and recipes and is your bonus at the end of this book.

As you can see, there are many choices for adding the relaxing properties to your bath. You can add in loose herbs to your bath, but will have herb clean up when you add it this way. There are herb bags that you can purchase or use a small piece of cheese cloth or material around your herbs, tying the bag or cloth tightly to hold herbs for easier clean up . Create many bags for lots of sweet floating smells in your tub!

There's oils, bubbling lotions and fizzing salts. Remember "Calgon, take me away!"? Those were fizzing salts that help to zap that tired feeling away. I will teach you how to make these bath time fun fizzes.

"Sorrow can be alleviated by good sleep, a bath and a glass of wine."

~Thomas Aquinas

Use the first bath recipe when you are tired, overworked and/or full of anxiety.

You will need a bath tub or a tub that you can soak your feet in. Fill your tub with hot water and add in cold water until you like the temperature. You can pick an oil or herb for this relaxing bath.

Herb Relaxing Bath

You will need a small cloth or material 2 to 3 inches in diameter or a herb bag. Add your herbs to the middle of your cloth or in your bag. Use a rubber band or ribbon to wrap the cloth closed and tie off.
Herb sacks have ties in them and work great.
1 tablespoon loose lavender herbs
2 tablespoon loose chamomile herbs
1/2 teaspoon sage leaves

Oil Relaxing Bath

This bath can be made straight into the bath water.
2 to 5 drops of lavender essential oils
2 to 5 drops of chamomile essential oils
1 drop sage essential oil

The following relaxing bath recipes work great when adding a relaxing drink like a cup of lavender and chamomile tea or a glass of red wine. While sitting in your relaxing bath, focus on your breathing, slowing it down and smoothing it out. Letting the belly rise and fall with each breath. All of these together will bring you to a state of complete relaxation.

As kids, we loved sitting in a bath with lots of bubbles. As adults, this feels like a luxury. Here is how you can make bubbles for your relaxing bath.

Relaxing Bubble Bath

You will need a small bowl, spoon, a funnel, and a bottle to put your bubble bath in.
1 cup of castile soap
¾ cup water
1 tablespoon vegetable glycerin

2 to 5 drops of lavender essential oils
2 to 5 drops of chamomile essential oils
1 drop sage essential oil

Place in order of listing in a small bowl and gently stir, careful not to make bubbles prematurely. Using a funnel, carefully pour the bubble bath into any empty bottle. Enjoy!

This bath goes great with a glass of wine, a Cosmopolitan, or if you really want to live it up, a glass of champagne!

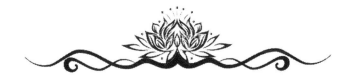

Relaxing baths are wonderful but at times we need something that will actually heal what ails us while soaking. These next recipes will heal many different issues.

Soothing Cough and Cold Bath
This bath can be made straight into the bath water.
Fill your bath with hot water, as hot as you can stand it.
4 to 7 drops of eucalyptus oil
2 drops of ravintsara oil
3 to 5 tablespoons mustard powder

This bath goes best with a cup of Gypsy Cold Tea or a tea to detox and immune boost. Soak in this bath while taking in deep breaths and focusing on clearing your lungs and breathing easier.

This next recipe's name does what it says it does! Use it as a foot bath when you have been on your feet all day or as a full bath when you have over worked your body.

Sore Muscle Relief Bath

This bath can be made straight into the bath water.
Fill your bath with hot water, as hot as you can stand it.
3 to 5 cups of Epsom salts
1 to 2 cups of mustard powder
1 drop of peppermint oil

Drink a glass of water with lemon with this bath or a replenishing drink.
Focus on breathing into sore spots or do the tub stretches you will find later in this chapter.

Use this next recipe when you feel the need to heal. This bath is good for cough, congestion or just plain healing of your body.

Herb Healing Bath

You will need small cloth or material 2 to 3 inches in diameter or an herb bag. Add your herbs to the middle of your cloth or in your bag. Use a rubber band or ribbon to wrap the cloth closed and tie off.
Herb sacks have ties in them and work great.
1/2 tablespoon eucalyptus leaves
1 tablespoon mustard powder
1/2 tablespoon wintergreen leaves
a pinch or two of rosemary leaves

This bath goes great with a hot tea that supports your issue. Use my Healing Pain and Illness guided meditation to help yourself heal.
This meditation teaches you how to breathe in green healing energy and the area in the body that needs healing on the inhale. On the exhale, release the pain or illness.

You can find the guided recording online or the written meditation in my The Key to Life is Balance book.

This next bath is fun to use!

Fizzing Bath Salts

You will need a bowl, a funnel, and a jar.
1 cup of Epsom salts
1 cup of sea salt
1 cup of baking soda (sifted)
1/2 cup of citric acid
Food color of your choice (if desired)
1 tablespoon skin safe fragrance oil of choice
Mix the Epsom salts, sea salt and baking soda together well, add a few drops of food color for desired color. Mix well. Add 1 tablespoon of skin safe fragrance oil. Mix well. Add 1/2 cup of citric acid. Mix well. Use a funnel to pour the fizzy salts mixture in a jar or container. Seal the jar or container. Decorate as desired. If giving away as a gift, add a label explaining what they are and how to use them. Use in warm water to get the maximum fizz.

There are times I want to take a hot bath in the AM before work. When I feel cold and need to warm up. I would choose a citrus bath to give me energy or a bath to help in getting me grounded. Now that you know how to make a bubble bath and fizzing baths, you can add the scents in these next bath soaks to the above bubble bath and fizzing recipes. When taking an energy soak, I like to stretch and massage my feet. You can do many stretches in the bath and I have listed my favorites here in this chapter.

Citrus Energy Soak

This bath can be made straight into the bath water.
Fill your bath with hot water, as hot as you can stand it.
2 drops Jasmine oil
1 drop peppermint oil
3 drops blood orange, orange or lemon
1 to 3 cups Epsom salts

Drinking coffee or some black tea will get you started for your day.

Here are some of the tub stretches I do when I need to add Yoga to my bath. It is a great way to incorporate my two favorites -
baths and Yoga.

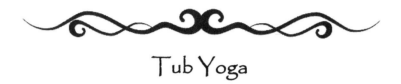

Tub Yoga

Neck Rotations - drop your chin to your chest and take in a deep cleansing breath. Then, rotate to the left for 3 to 5 turns, breathing into the rotations and working to gain more movement with each turn. Repeat 3 to 5 rotations, now to the right. Do until relaxation and better range of motion is achieved.

Neck Stretch - drop your head to the right and hold, let the left shoulder fall away, like having a tug of war with your neck and opposite shoulder. Repeat with the other side, hold stretch for 15 to 25 counts.

Shoulder Rolls - open up your chest by lifting the breast bone up and then rotate your shoulders back and around, 6 to 8 times. Breathing from the belly and working to gain more movement in the shoulders with each turn.

Forward fold - sitting in the bath with legs extended, lift up through the breast bone on an inhale, and exhale folding at your hips. Hold on to your feet if you can reach them. Hold this stretch for 15 counts. Repeat 2 or 3 times.

Waist twist - same sitting position, lift up through the breast bone, inhale, and exhale twisting your torso as you hold onto the side of the tub. Hold stretch for 15 counts and repeat on the other side.

I would like to take a moment to explain a bit about Grounding. Being grounded simply means you are connected to the Earth, and the Earth then can give you energy. It is like plugging in to an energy circuit. Sometimes we feel like things are not going right. If you feel you are not in balance, I always suggest focusing on getting Grounded as the first step. It is always best to do some sort of Grounding ritual every day to make sure you are always plugged in. You can find more about Grounding, and how to Ground in my first book. For the next Spa-Cipe, just know that being grounded will give you more energy and help you feel supported and secure.

Grounding Bath

This bath can be made straight into the bath water.
Fill your bath with hot water, as hot as you can stand it.
1 drop Sandalwood oil
1 drop Sage oil
2 cups Epsom salts

This bath goes well with a glass of calcium bentonite clay, a Kombucha drink or a drink that will replenish your energy.

Find two dark or black rocks in your yard or better yet by a river. I use black rocks in meditation to help take away negative energy and to get grounded. I keep a set of two black rocks by my bed, by all my sinks and in my car. I use them to do a recharge and to cleanse my energy.
When I worked at the local drug rehab I would teach a meditation using these rocks. This meditation is perfect for a Grounding Bath.

"The foot feels the foot
when it feels the ground."
~Buddha

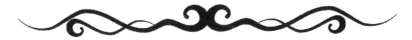

Grounding Meditation

Place a black rock in both hands while sitting in your Grounding Bath. Start by taking in three deep belly breaths. Inhale and let the belly rise, taking your time with this inhale. Exhale letting the belly fall. Keep up this deep belly breathing until you start to feel relaxed. Holding each of the rocks in your hands, feel them and roll them in your palms, thinking and feeling gratitude. Thank the black rocks for taking away anything that no longer serves you. Thank them for soaking up any negativity you may be holding onto or that was picked up during your day. Keep thanking the rocks (which come from the Earth) for taking away any and all negative energy from your body as you roll them in your palms. Sit quietly, rolling the rocks in your palms, feeling grateful and sending negative energy to the rocks. Start to think about what you are grateful for and if any negative thoughts come to you, send them to the rocks. Stay with this until you feel like coming back to reality or your water starts to get cold. Cleanse rocks with sage oil or a lighted sage stick after each use.

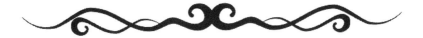

Feeling itchy, have a skin irritation or feel like you need a good old fashioned detox? This bath is not only relaxing but it will detox your skin removing impurities and restoring the proper pH levels of your skin and body.
It also goes well with the pH Balance drink on the next page. The ingredients in this drink will cure bouts of gout, joint pain, and put your pH back into balance.

Detox Bath

This bath can be made straight into the bath water.
Fill your bath with hot water, as hot as you can stand it.
2 cups Epsom salts
1 teaspoon baking soda
3 to 5 tablespoons calcium bentonite clay
squeeze in some lemon, and 1 drop Lavender

Soak in this bath for 15 to 20 mins, you can do the Grounding Meditation if you want. Focus on letting go and detoxing your mind and body in this bath.

pH Balance drink
8 oz of warm water
1 tablespoon apple cider vinegar
1 teaspoon baking soda
substitution - swap apple cider vinegar
with the juice of two lemons.

Finally, for you shower people, here are some Spa-Cipes for your shower. You can make these with any scented oil you wish, like lavender to make it a relaxing shower, or citrus to make it a energy boosting shower. If you have a cold, congestion or cough, making this next recipe will totally help. Throwing one of these shower soothers into your shower will clear your airways fast, helping you breathe easy again.
They are so simple to make as well – you just need baking soda, water and essential oils!

Shower Soothers

You will need a bowl, muffin tin,
muffin liners and a oven.
1 cup baking soda
1/3 cup + 2 tablespoons water
4 to 6 drops of rosemary essential oil
6 to 8 drops of eucalyptus essential oil
2 drops of lavender essential oil
1 drop peppermint essential oil

Stir together the baking soda and water into a thick
paste, the thicker the better. About 1 cup of baking
soda to 1/3 of a cup of water. Add more baking soda if
it needs thickening. Fill each muffin cup halfway. Add
a few generous drops of each of the essential oils. Then
fill each muffin cup (using liners works best) up with
the rest of the 'cold batter'. Bake for 20 minutes at 350
degrees. Let cool completely before removing them
from the pan/liners. Once cooled, add a few more
generous drops of each essential oil to both the top &
the bottom of the soothers. Store them in a airtight
container up to 6 months, add the essential oils to both
sides about 5 minutes before using them. Put the disc in
the bottom of the shower in front of your toes in your
hot shower. These can also be placed in a bowl with
boiling water with a towel placing it over your head
and breathe in for relief of cough, colds and congestion.

The smells are important in your space. Holistic room sprays are very easily made and give you all of the creative control.

Room Sprays

You will need a spray bottle.
Fill bottle 3/4 full of distilled water,
add 5 to 8 drops of any essential oils
Combine scents if you like.
Spray your sheets, the dog blanket and the bathroom.

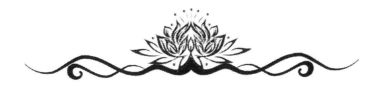

Money Attraction Spray

You will need a spray bottle.
Fill bottle 3/4 full of distilled water,
add 1 to 3 drops each Vetiver, Frankincense and Myrrh.
Spray on yourself when you want money to come in.
Place on a cotton ball and blot on out going checks,
cash and bills to send that energy right back to you.
Open your mind to the abundance of
money flowing to you now!

I wish you much Love, Success and Abundance!
~The Groovy Goddess

Chapter Three
Food Facials

Now that you have the soothing soaks to play with, you are ready for my signature food facial recipes and the wonderfully effective facial treatments. These are Spa-Cipes you can enjoy while in your relaxing baths to get the full spa effect.

    Before I go into the Food Facials and the Spa-Cipes for them, I want to give you some background on how to mix all of these wonderful ingredients. When I first started out, I used a small food processor to mix. It worked ok, but not great. Food processors don't create a creamy smooth mask, as you will be left with small chunks of food. The masks will still work, but it is a bit messy. I bought a Vita-Mix this past year and now my food facials come out creamy and smooth every time. Find what works for you, but a high speed blender is your best bet to get the best mask possible.

"The beauty of a woman is not in a facial mode but the true beauty in a woman is reflected in her soul. It is the caring that she lovingly gives the passion that she shows. The beauty of a woman grows with the passing years."

~Audrey Hepburn

This is the very first food facial mask I made. It will help with acne and get rid of excess oils in your skin. But first, here's a sweet trick to cleanse your face!

Honey

That's right, Honey! It can be used daily as a facial cleanser. It does an excellent job of cleaning and moisturizing, making skin soft and smooth and it works with every skin type!

To wash your face with honey: For make-up free skin, squirt a small amount of honey (less than a teaspoon) into the palm of your hand. Rub the honey between your palms with a little warm water and then massage into your face. Wash off with warm water.

To remove make up with honey: pour a small amount of honey onto a wet wash cloth and sprinkle with a little baking soda. Use the washcloth to wash the face. Remove any residue with warm water.

For dry skin: mix a little milk or cream with honey for a cleanser.

For extremely oily skin: try adding a little lemon juice to the honey.

Honey can enhance your beauty routine in many ways, including being used as a hair treatment. Go ahead and add it to any of the Hair Spa-Cipes.

Oatmeal Facial

You will need a bowl, face towel and
face paint brush.
1/2 cup cooked oatmeal
1 egg (whites only)

Mix these two ingredients to create a thick paste. Place a hot towel on your face and leave it there for a minute or two. This is relaxing and will help open pores so the mask can work deeply.
Use the honey for washing your face. Brush on mask with a face paint brush and leave on for 10 to 15 minutes. This mask will dry and feel like it is pulling. Use a hot towel to take off the mask by using an upward motion as you wipe.

My all time favorite facial is Pumpkin because you can use it for most skin types. Although I have been doing these food facials since I was a kid, I never tried pumpkin until later in my 30's.

I was in massage school and one of the girls in my class was already an esthetician and invited me to do a trade. She gave me a pumpkin facial. The smell was amazing! It gave me a warm comfortable feeling and my skin did look and feel great. This was my first real facial I would experience and it did teach me a lot about giving facials to others.

I was in love! Her pumpkin facial was a product with chemicals in it, but I knew I could mix up some real pumpkin and have a pie smelling mask people will love.

Food not only feeds us from the inside but it can act as nourishment on the outside as well. You can literally watch the skin soaking up the food as it disappears on the face.

The food facials I make for the spa are simple and effective and I have been offering them for about seven years; they are pumpkin, tomato/cucumber, banana and avocado. I love to add chocolate to the avocado from Valentine's Day on through the Summer because chocolate actually helps protect the skin from sun damage and pollution, too.

As I write this, I have a banana mask on my face. It's the best stuff in the world for breakouts! I add comfrey gel to this facial to help calm down the breakouts while the banana heals them.

The tomato and cucumber mask is a great way to heal wrinkles and slow down the aging process. Cucumbers hydrate and tomatoes have lycopene, which is an antioxidant and works as a sunscreen from within. These antioxidants make tomato an anti-aging product as they help in fighting cellular damage and reddening of skin.

The chocolate and avocado mask helps to add oils back in the face and protects skin from damage. You will notice the chocolate facial and chocolate pudding recipe in Chapter Nine are similar.

I was at a raw food workshop and the presenter made this chocolate pudding from avocados that tasted exactly like chocolate pudding. While making this one day, I realized all the ingredients were good for the skin and I used some of it as a facial. I had my Valentine's Day special and it is still a hit every year. The recipe in this chapter is not one you can eat as it does add in the aloe products but not the agave for taste. The chocolate pudding recipe is located in the Balance Cleanse in Chapter Nine.

I don't always do my food facials during bath and relaxing time. I do them first thing in the morning while doing my morning routine. If I wake up and I find a breakout, I go to the fridge and get out my banana mask or go get my clay mixture. Even though food facials are fast and easy to make, you can have some on hand in your fridge. When you pre-make food facials they will last a couple of days to a couple of weeks in the fridge, depending on which ones you are making. My recipes will make 4 to 5 masks at a time. If you want to just make a mask for one or two treatments, I suggest cutting them in half.

My signature food facials that I mix up at my spa have a base powder and aloe liquid that come from a product line I use. This company is Set N Me Free from Oregon. The base product is natural and helps me to create a professional grade product from food and herbs.

I first learned about Set N Me Free from a local esthetician. She was closing her location and contacted me about product she wanted to sell. I liked the natural ingredients right away, made mostly of aloe and in gels, lotions and liquids. Aloe is a healing plant and heals the skin fast. But, all the aloe you find in the stores are a gel and are very sticky and the lotions have other ingredients I do not want on my skin.

I signed up to take a workshop on how to use these aloe products and the first thing they did was hand out a recipe book. The instructor said, "You can add food to our product to enhance the effectiveness and create amazing professional grade spa treatments." I was hooked! I could now offer high grade signature facials when I used the aloe product as a base.

Set N Me Free is sold to spa wholesalers only. You can purchase the base product online through a spa dealer, like myself. You can then add it to the following recipes to recreate what I make at Balance Studio Spa. If using Set N Me Free Aloe Vera products follow the instructions on the packaging and add to any of these recipes.

The following recipes are wonderful as food alone and they are very effective on the skin! Remember, you can be creative and add in other food and herbs!

Set N Me Free product listing that I use:

Masking Powder - this is a powder that will enhance your mask and helps to keep your ingredients together, while giving the mask extra healing for your skin. Ingredients are corn starch, honey, aloe, witch hazel, borage, stone root, elder flower and blueberry oil.

Masking Liquid - this is a liquid and is aloe with some ginseng and blueberry oil. You can substitute using aloe water or coconut water in your mask.

Comfrey Gel - aloe, comfrey, retinyl palmitate (vitamin A), tocopheryl (vitamin E oil), eucalyptus globulus oil, clove oil, peppermint oil. (I love this gel and have not found anything like it on the market.)

Aloe Toner - aloe, witch hazel

I will now go over my signature food only facials that I use at my spa. The following is a step by step process of how I apply each mask and create the 3 mask food facials with eye treatment. The first mask I apply to clients is the Clay Mask to detox the skin. You will learn more about this wonderful clay in Chapter Nine. It can be used topically to detox the skin and heal many skin problems, to heal acne, rashes and bug bites. This is my *go to* mask to heal anything and everything wrong with my skin. I brush on the clay mask, let it dry for a bit and then steam the clay into the skin. FYI...the clay may make the irritation look redder for the first 24 hours and this is because it is pulling out the deeply set in toxins.

Stick with it, as that will change during the 24 hour period and will start looking much better fast. I like to start my facials off with the clay mask because pulling out toxins is always the best place to start.

Clay Mask

You will need a bowl, a plastic spoon (using plastic when spooning out clay is recommended) and a face paint brush. Do not mix this mask in a blender or processor.
1 teaspoon calcium bentonite clay
1 tablespoon aloe, coconut or plain water
2 to 3 drops of apple cider vinegar (if you are having bad breakouts or a facial rash)

Mix the water and clay into a paste that is smooth and thick. It is best to mix the clay and let it sit for 30 minutes to thicken up. Place a hot towel on your face and leave it there for a minute or two. This is relaxing and will help open pores so the mask can work deeply. Wash face and neck with honey and then rinse. Brush on mask with a face paint brush and leave on for 10 to 15 minutes. This mask will dry and feel like it is pulling. Some say it feels like a itching or burning sensation. If that sensation is too much, take the mask off. You may experience redness in areas that needed detox. The redness will go away after a few minutes.

Use a hot towel to take off the clay mask and use a upward motion as you wipe. Apply next mask or moisturizer. You may use the clay mask weekly or twice a day on a problem area like acne or a rash . Be careful of over drying your skin as this mask is very effective.

This clay mask is a better way to clear up poison oak, helps with bug bites and is an effective way to treat eczema and psoriasis.

Next up is a nourishing mask. I love this next mask at Fall time, not only because I love pumpkin *everything* during this time of year, but also when I heat this up and it smells just like pumpkin pie. Pumpkin nourishes skin as it contains vitamin A, alpha and beta-carotenes, vitamins C, K, and E, plus minerals, including magnesium, potassium, and iron. These ingredients will help in balancing out the skin and you will love the look and feel of your face.

Pumpkin Mask

You will need a bowl, face towel and face paint brush.
Mixed best in a high speed blender or processor.
1 cup uncooked or canned (organic) pumpkin
1 teaspoon coconut oil (melted)
1 teaspoon comfrey gel or loose comfrey herbs
1 tablespoon aloe, coconut or plain water
3 to 4 mint leaves
(to help reduce dark circles under the eyes)

Blend ingredients together until creamy and smooth.
Place a hot towel on your face and leave it there for a
minute or two. This is relaxing and will help open
pores so the mask can work deeply. Wash face and
neck with honey, or use as the second mask after clay
mask. This mask can be brushed onto face and neck or
massaged into skin with clean fingers, covering face
and neck. Leave on 15 to 20 minutes, place a hot towel
on your face for 2 minutes and wipe off in an upward
direction.

This next facial mask will hydrate and replenish. I
use this mask on aging and dry skin. Tomatoes are
great for the skin as they have cooling and
astringent properties to them.

They are rich in vitamin C, brightening dull skin, along with vitamin A, which is needed for healthy skin. It's naturally acidic so it helps balance the skin and get rid of excessive oil. The many antioxidants in tomatoes help depleted skin. Cucumber is hydrating and helps to replenish moisture in your skin.

They have the same pH as the skin so they help restore the protective acid mantle–they also possess hydrating, nourishing and astringent properties. The skin of a cucumber is rich in fiber and contains a variety of beneficial minerals including silica, potassium and magnesium. The silica in cucumber is an essential component of healthy connective tissue, which includes muscles, tendons, ligaments, cartilage, and bone. Cucumber juice is often recommended as a source of silica to improve the complexion and health of the skin, plus it's naturally hydrating—a must for glowing skin.

Tomato and Cucumber Mask

You will need a bowl, face towel and
face paint brush.
This mask is best mixed in a high speed blender.
1/2 cup cucumber
One small tomato
2 tablespoons coconut oil
1 tablespoon aloe or plain water

Blend ingredients together until creamy and smooth.
These ingredients are watery, and you can add more
coconut oil to thicken it up or add in more masking
powder. Place a hot towel on your face and leave it
there for a minute or two, this is relaxing and will help
open pores so the mask can work deeply. Wash face
and neck with honey, or use as the second mask after
clay mask. This mask can be brushed onto face and
neck or massaged into skin with clean fingers, covering
face and neck. Leave on 15 to 20 minutes, place a hot
towel on your face for 2 minutes and wipe off in an
upward direction.

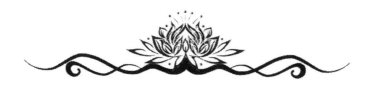

This mask will help clear up acne and tone down red blotchy skin. Banana as a daily treatment can be used just by rubbing the banana peel onto the skin, the riper, the better.

Banana Mask

You will need a bowl, face towel and face paint brush. This mask is best mixed in a high speed blender or processor.
1/2 banana- riper is better
One tbsp comfrey gel or loose herbs(if desired)
1 tablespoon aloe or plain water

Blend ingredients together until creamy and smooth. Place a hot towel on your face and leave it there for a minute or two, this is relaxing and will help open pores so the mask can work deeply. Wash face and neck with honey, or use as the second mask after clay mask. This mask can be brushed onto face and neck or massaged into skin with clean fingers, covering face and neck. Leave on 15 to 20 minutes, place a hot towel on your face for 2 minutes and wipe off in an upward direction

Avocado Mask

You will need a bowl, face towel and
face paint brush. This mask is best mixed in a high
speed blender or processor.
1/2 avocado skinned and mashed
1 tablespoon aloe or plain water
1 teaspoon coconut oil
1 teaspoon honey
1 to 2 teaspoons unsweetened chocolate powder (to
make the chocolate facial)

Blend ingredients together until creamy and smooth.
Place a hot towel on your face and leave it there for a
minute or two, this is relaxing and will help open pores
so the mask can work deeply. Wash face and neck with
your favorite face wash. Or use as the second mask
after clay mask. This mask can be brushed onto face
and neck or massaged into skin with clean fingers,
covering face and neck. Leave on 15 to 20 minutes,
place a hot towel on your face for 2 minutes and then
wipe off in an upward direction.

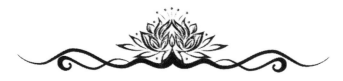

The last mask I use for my signature food facial is
this one. It is a skin toner and it will tighten skin,
too.

Egg White Toner Mask

You will need a bowl and cotton pad or face paint brush. This mask can be runny, so I use a cotton round pad (not cotton ball) to apply it. You can brush it on, too.

1 egg white
1 teaspoon witch hazel
1 teaspoon apple cider vinegar

Soak the cotton pad in this mixture and use it to apply to the skin. Leave it on until it dries and remove with a cold towel. Cold water will help to close down the open pores. After you are done with your masks, add your favorite moisturizer. The mask recipes given here can be used weekly to keep your skin looking its best. The clay mask can be used a couple of times a day on spots you are healing, just be mindful not to dry out these spots.

Next, I will give you some wonderful things you can add to the facial recipes that heal and help with other skin issues.

- Add in mint for relief of dark circles under the eyes.
- Lemon will help to even out skin color as it acts as a skin bleach.
- A squeeze or two of an orange to get Vitamin C on the skin to help heal dark spots from sun damage.
- Add in honey to exfoliate, increase elasticity, balance out oily skin, stimulate collagen production, and minimize lines and wrinkles.
- Coconut oil - I can't say enough about this wonder food. Just applying coconut oil to your skin at night will give your skin a healthy treat.
- Apple Cider Vinegar - use this as an astringent after working in the yard or sweating. It will clean pores of dirt that may cause a buildup. I use it after I wash my face two to three times a week.

Try this trick to help with puffy eyes and this treatment will also help eliminate dark circles under the eye.

Cucumber and Mint Eye Treatment
You will need a bowl, face paint brush or round cotton pads.

1/4 cup cut cucumber
5 to 8 mint leaves
1/4 cup water/aloe water or coconut water
Blend ingredients, pour in a small bowl and add two round cotton pads. Let the pads soak up the goodness and place on your eyes during your bath or while relaxing. Re-soak until all ingredients are gone. Or you can brush the treatment below your eyes and leave on while you relax.

Use the following facial mask if you are prone to skin cancers or have a skin cancer you are dealing with. You can use this mask on ringworm or serious skin conditions.

Turmeric Face Mask

You will need a bowl, mixing spoon,
facial paint brush, and towel.
1 teaspoon ground turmeric
2 teaspoons oatmeal
1/2 teaspoon coconut oil (melted)
3 tablespoons plain yogurt
(or sour cream, cream, or milk)
1 teaspoon Vitamin E oil

Heat up your coconut oil to liquidfy, mix all ingredients together. After using a gentle face wash, brush this mask on to your face and skin. Making sure you completely cover problem areas. Leave on for 20 minutes. Wash off with warm water. The turmeric will stain clothing and towel but not your skin.

I add a sugar scrub to my facials after the second mask to help in removal of dead skin and to exfoliate at a deep level. My recipe also helps to add oils as you exfoliate. There are many options as to the oil used.

Facial Sugar Scrub

You will need a bowl
1 teaspoon coconut sugar (or any sugar)
2 teaspoons olive, hemp or avocado oil
1 drop of lavender essential oil

With clean fingers, scoop up the mixture and start to rub vigorously in small circles in a upward motion on face, neck and chest. Careful not to damage skin; be effective and gentle at the same time.

The Alpha-Hydroxy Acid that is found in papaya has beneficial anti-aging properties.

Wrinkle and Skin

Whitener Treatment

1 Papaya (eat the papaya and use the skin)
Rub the papaya on the skin and leave on for 5 minutes.
Wash off with cold water.
I would use this treatment alone or after the second mask and after the scrub exfoliate.
Do not leave on any longer as it may dry out your freshly hydrated skin.

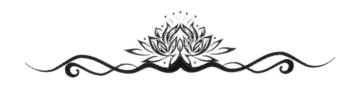

To add hydration to your skin after your food facial, here is a lotion you make into bars. To apply lotion to your skin, just rub it on the face in an upward motion to release the goodness on to your skin. Until you get your bars made, you can simply scoop up some coconut oil with your clean fingers and apply to the face.

This next Spa-Cipe makes a great gift idea especially if you make them in molds that have fun shapes or cut them into small bars and wrap them with a pretty cloth.

Natural Face Lotion Bars

You will need a double boiler, spoon,
and a pan to be your mold.
1 cup coconut oil
1 cup shea, cocoa or mango butter
1 cup beeswax
1 drop lavender
1 drop chamomile

Bring water to a boil. Stir ingredients constantly until they are melted and smooth:
Remove from heat and add the essential oils.
Gently stir by hand until essential oils are incorporated.

Carefully pour into molds or whatever you will be
allowing the lotion bars to harden in.

I choose the lavender and chamomile for their relaxing
properties. The choices are endless! Here are a couple
more:

For those of you that need a more even skin tone, add a
couple of drops of real lemon juice (add pulp for a nice
textured look).

If you tend to have some redness or rosacea add a drop
or two of comfrey oil.

I learned a new trick from Facebook the other
day and it worked great! It is not a Spa-Cipe for skin or
face, but a face lift for your furniture. I recently bought
a nice looking hutch from Craigslist. My partner does
have a knack for finding the best things on Craigslist,
and he was wanting to sand it down and refinish it.
That just overwhelms me because it is a lot of work and
I do have a book to write. I did this instead...

Use this on wood furniture that needs cleaning,
has scratches or knicks.

Facelift for your Furniture

You will need a jar and dusting cloth.
1 cup Canola oil (I use Olive oil)
1/4 cup white vinegar

Place ingredients in the jar to store or use right away.
Dip your dusting cloth in the mixture and wipe down
your wood piece. The scratches will disappear before
your eyes. Nicks will fill in and blend with the wood,
you will almost not know they are there. It will clean
off grime and dust from your furniture, too
. It is just like giving your wood and home a facelift.
Add some lemon or orange essential oils if you want
that clean citrus smell throughout your home.

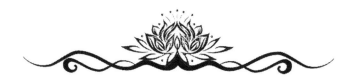

Chapter Four
Detox Wraps

I have struggled with weight issues my whole life. Through all the diets, up and downs of weight gains and losses, I was never introduced to body wraps until I finally felt like I had the weight thing licked. I am open minded, but I also have a skeptical side. I need to be shown that something works before I believe it and tell others about it.

I was not a believer until that Set N Me Free workshop. I insisted I be the one wrapped, and then I could check it out first hand. I was told to wear a bathing suit under my clothes and be ready to be in it and wrapped in front of 25 or so strangers. I was excited, not only to have a new treatment I could offer at the spa, but to learn about ways to help my body be better, too. There was some fear creeping up about being in a bathing suit in front of all these strangers. As always, to get where I needed and wanted to be, I needed to push past that fear.

Before I was to be wrapped, they measured and marked me with a sharpie where the tape measure was to get an accurate reading of my inch loss. It came time for me to be wrapped and I was a bit nervous. I am claustrophobic and when they started to wrap me and were talking about cocooning me in blankets, I thought, "Hey am I going to freak out? "

I did not freak out but it was a very odd feeling to me. I usually do not lay on my back for very long and 45 minutes wrapped like a mummy cocooned in blankets on my back is too much for me. Even today I have to lay on my side in a wrap.

I let my clients know that if they have a problem with feeling confined to move to where they feel comfortable while in the wrap. There is nothing you can really do that will make the wrap not work for you other than getting out of it before the recommended time is up. I had one client that jumped out of the wrap after only fifteen minutes because she could not lay still and thought the wrap would still work after only that short of time. This client had a hard time giving relaxation to herself.

In the wrap I was feeling an itch type of feeling all over my body and I was told that is normal. It is the wrap actively moving the herbs through the blood stream. It came time for the unwrapping and I saw the mouths of the people watching drop. "They could see a difference?" I thought. Then, they measured me and I was twenty inches smaller all over. I did have to run to the bathroom shortly after they unwrapped me. When I put back on my clothes I felt smaller especially in the belly area. My skin felt amazingly soft and hydrated.

I know now why they saw a difference and this is what I tell my weight loss clients. Losing the weight is not the only focus. Changing the texture of your skin helps you to see the difference. I know from firsthand experience when losing weight, you may still see bumps on the legs (cellulite) and dry skin that makes you still feel fat. Treating the skin while losing weight helps you to see the differences. Skin also needs to be treated to tighten. I know many people that lost the weight and hate their bodies still, because they did not do anything about tightening the skin and now have hanging skin in places. This is why I recommend doing body treatments to treat your skin. When your skin is hydrated and when cellulite is removed from the legs and hips you can see a big difference. This will help you to start loving your body.

If you are going to give yourself a body wrap always give yourself the time to do it. Body wraps do work when you let them. Basically it is the same concept as drinking a smoothie with herbs that detox. A greater benefit of having a body wrap is that you will get a skin treatment detox and get relaxation all at the same time. Now who doesn't need or want a full body skin treatment and some relaxation? The herbs soak into the pores while you are cocooned and relaxed and then go into the blood stream just as if you drank the herbs. The herbs then go to work detoxing you from the inside out.

Seven years ago, when I began giving and doing body wraps on myself, I did not really understand what the herbs could do for the body. I have since learned a lot, and understand why and how these wraps work.

I had a friend tell me once that I do treatments like Edgar Cayce. I did not know who this man was. I started to research him and I found that my treatments were starting to look like things he did to heal people. Edgar Cayce was a intuitive healer that was far before the times of New Age. He was alive from 1877 until 1945 and his story began with a healing of himself from a local Hypnotherapist. He then started to heal people by meditating on their names and location from letters they would send. One of his treatments was wrapping parts of the body with cloths soaked in castor oil. After discovering this, I was convinced that I was on the right path in adding body wraps to my life.

I do not make my detox wraps, as I get the gel and concentrate liquid from Set N Me Free. I trust the formula that this company has come up with because I have seen seven years of results on myself and with clients. Here are the active ingredients found in the gel:

- Aloe Water
- Guar Gum
- Saffron
- Lady Slipper
- Chickweed
- Papaya
- Kelp
- Cleavers
- Chaparral
- Parsley
- Hawthorne Berry

The solution of highly active concentrates will tone and tighten surface skin and boost cellular activity to restore elasticity and firmness to the tissues. Natural aromas benefit the body through inter-cellular osmosis to produce positive therapeutic effects. Toxins are eliminated naturally through the lymphatic system. The treatment is safe for anyone as no dehydration or compression is used.

The Set N Me Free company has two forms of wraps. The one I use at the spa with heated wraps, and one that is a gel that you brush on and then cover with plastic wrap. While in the plastic wrap you can put on warm clothing or get under warm blankets for 45 minutes. This treatment is great for sunburned skin because it is cold and this treatment is easily done at home.

I have given myself the hot wraps many times and it is very hard to do yourself. It is difficult to wrap yourself and get cocooned under blankets. You end up being cold and not getting the full relaxation you can get if someone is doing the wrap for you. If you want to start getting detox wraps at home, I do suggest getting the gel from a spa dealer and then you have full control of doing the wraps yourself and it is more cost effective.

You can try your hand at mixing the potion yourself. Play with the amounts of each of the ingredients into the aloe water. Place the ingredients in about 8 to 10 cups of water and heat 9 to 10 rolls of cloth in the heating mix for 45 minutes. Then, wrap yourself like a mummy and cocoon yourself in blankets for 45 mins. Take off the cloths and then go about your day. DO NOT shower for 24 hours to allow the ingredients to soak in fully!

Remember after a detox wrap you should drink 3-4 liters of water during the 24-hour period following the treatment. It will flush toxins through the system to ensure that the size loss will stay off. I tell clients to keep up the drinking of water for several days after and remember, you are detoxing. If you get a headache, emotional, or feel under the weather in the days following your wrap, keep drinking water! These symptoms will subside as you flush your system.

If you would like to research this more and check out informative videos about body wraps, go to:
www.SetNMeFree.com.

Chapter Five
Healing Body Treatments

About 85% of my massage clients have dry skin and tell me their skin is dry. Even the people that say they apply lotion say their skin is dry. I feel the skin needs treatments and most of the lotions have man-made chemical ingredients in them. These ingredients take away hydration and dry out the skin even more.
Skin treatments are left on the skin longer than it would take for you to apply lotion. This length of time helps build up layers of hydration and gives time for those layers to deeply soak in.

Leaving the oils and food in these recipes on your skin for at least 30 to 45 minutes will not only give you the relaxation you seek but the skin treatment you will love.

I have clients tell me they use nothing on their skin and those that use nothing tend to have really dry skin. Hydration in the body is important in many ways to skin care. Proper hydration in the body helps the body assimilate essential nutrients, excrete toxins, assists in maintaining pH balances, and decreases chances of constipation and urinary infections. As far as the skin itself is concerned, it reduces the signs of aging, keeps skin soft and helps to hold on to elasticity. The water content in skin helps it perform its protective functions.

With proper hydration, skin looks firm and supple, and is able to heal faster when injured. If dermal cells are not hydrated properly, they lose suppleness and hair follicles can get blocked, causing bacterial accumulation. Good hydration can help in the treatment of acne, too.

When skin is not adequately hydrated, it loses thickness, and offers less body protection. Skin tone becomes dry and dull, and extra sensitive. Wrinkles are formed easily. Diabetics should be particularly careful to keep well hydrated.

Drinking plenty of water is a great place to start and getting a body treatment is the best step forward you can take in learning about loving your body. Texture is half the battle in changing your body image. I hear many times women say they need to lose weight and I look at them and they don't look over weight to me. It is the cellulite on the legs and hips that makes women feel fat.

Cellulite is toxins that are stuck in the soft fat cells of the body. Moving those toxins out of the legs will make the legs look smoother and this will give you more confidence. I know this one first hand because I have finally rid my legs of cellulite. I remember looking at my legs after losing weight, and I still thought they were fat. Now I think, "Hey, I look good when I look in the mirror!"

My skin is very important to me. I take very good care of it. Body treatments will give you confidence and a new found Love for yourself.

Use this treatment for dry skin, after being in the sun too long (not burned) and when you want to do something lovely for yourself.

Avocado and Egg Treatment

You will need a bowl, body paint brush, a thermal blanket or large plastic blanket, several warm blankets and some hand towels or a bath towel.

Prepare your place to relax by laying out the warm blankets and then the plastic or thermal blanket on top.

2 avocados (skinned and pitted)
2 eggs whole
1 large or 3 small tomatoes
1 orange slice squeezed (eat the rest of the orange)
1/2 cup olive oil
1 cup aloe water

Mix all ingredients in the blender. Place mixed ingredients in the bowl. Stand on a towel next to your place of rest and paint the mixture on your body. Paint in a upward direction towards the heart. Make sure to cover all areas that you feel really need it.

After covering your body with the mixture, lay in the center of the blankets and carefully wrap yourself in. Have a timer set to watch your time and just relax. If you love to read, you can keep enough of your hands and arms out of the wrap to hold your book or Kindle.

After the time is up, unwrap yourself, and shower off or soak in a bath for up to 5 minutes and then shower off. After drying off, you'll want to apply moisturizer. Only apply one that will not dehydrate you again. I suggest a straight coconut oil.

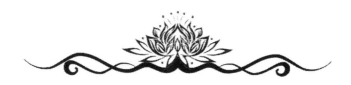

Use this next recipe when you are suffering from hives, eczema or psoriasis.

Clay, Coconut Oil and More Treatment

You will need a bowl, body paint brush, and a large bath or beach towel. Prepare your place to relax by laying out your towel to sit on.
1/2 cup to 1 cup calcium bentonite clay
(depending on how much skin you are treating)
1 cup coconut oil
1/4 cup hot water
1/2 tablespoon apple cider vinegar
1 tablespoon honey
1 tablespoon vitamin E oil
1 tablespoon comfrey gel or loose herb

If skin is extremely itchy, cut the clay from 1 cup to 1/2 a cup or from 1/2 a cup to a 1/4 of a cup and add in 1/2 a cup oatmeal.

Add clay, coconut oil and hot water mix in blender. The hot water will melt the coconut oil.
Add the rest of the ingredients and blend. Apply to areas as needed and let sit up to 45 minutes while you relax on your towel. Read a book, check out an old movie or meditate while you wait.

Use this treatment when you are going to spend time out in the sun or as a pre summer treatment. Chocolate protects skin from the sun damage and antioxidants help with aging of skin.

Chocolate and Clay Treatment

You will need a bowl, body paint brush, a thermal blanket or large plastic blanket, several warm blankets and some hand towels or a bath towel. Prepare your place to relax by laying out the warm blankets and then the plastic or thermal blanket on top.

1/2 cup calcium bentonite clay
3 tablespoons of Cocoa powder
mix in aloe water until powder is a
consistency of a paste
you may double recipe if you want a thicker layer
on your skin or better coverage.

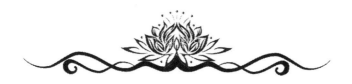

If you find yourself with a case of poison oak, ring worm, or acne use just the clay as a paste.

Calcium Bentonite Clay Paste

You will need a bowl and face or body paint brush.
2 to 4 tablespoons calcium bentonite clay
Mix with aloe, coconut or regular water until paste.
Brush on affected area and let stand for 15 to 20 mins.
Do this three times a day. Your rash will dry up usually within 48 hours.

What kind of massage therapist would I be if I did not give you an easy to make massage oil or cream? The most simple way is to use coconut oil but here are two versions that have a great smell and are Divine to apply! It's also great as a gift when placed in a decorative bottle.

Massage Oil

You will need a bowl, a mixing spoon, and a colored glass jar (oils keep better in colored glass jars stored in a cool dry place).

You will start with a vegetable base oil to be your carrier oil. Then select your essential oils. There are so many choices here.

- **Avocado oil** -An excellent carrier oil for those with mature skin, or conditions that require special care. Re-hydrates and nourishes sun dried skin, and is easily absorbed.

- **Almond oil** - Very moisturizing, rich in essential fatty acids and vitamins A & E. Light both in odor and color and while it is suitable for all skin types, is particularly useful for dry or sensitive skin.

- **Apricot Kernel** - Similar to Sweet Almond oil chemically, but with a wonderfully light consistency and aroma making it particularly suitable for facial massage and treatments.

- **Grapeseed oil** - a light, gentle, emollient oil with a low odor and good penetration. Readily absorbed by the skin and carries a low risk of allergy. Especially popular with professional massage therapists.

- **Hazelnut oil -** Has no taste or smell to overpower other fragrances. It penetrates deeply, and has great moisturizing capacity.

- **Jojoba oil** - Not an oil , but a liquid wax, with natural moisturizing and healing properties, suitable for all skin types. Like grape seed oil, it is not a nut oil, so it's very suitable for those with sensitive skin.

- **Wheat germ oil** - renowned for its high content of Vitamin E, an antioxidant, as well as fatty acids and is particularly useful for dry or mature skin.

Here are just some of the fragrant essential oils you can add:

- Black Pepper oil
- Cinnamon oil
- Geranium oil
- Jasmine oil
- Lavender oil
- Orange oil
- Peppermint oil
- Rosewood oil
- Rose oil
- Sandalwood oil
- Ylang Ylang oil

Here are some variations to create the massage you'll Love!

Abundance of Flower

- 4 ounces of your preferred carrier oil
- 15 drops of rosewood oil
- 10 drops of geranium oil
- 8 drops of jasmine oil
- 3 drops of lavender oil

Grounding Scents

- 4 ounces of your preferred carrier oil
- 15 drops of sandalwood oil
- 9 drops of cinnamon oil
- 6 drops of peppermint oil
- 5 drops of black pepper oil

Creating Energy

- 4 ounces of your preferred carrier oil
- 15 drops of rose oil
- 15 drops of ylang ylang oil
- 10 drops of jasmine oil
- 2 drops of orange oil

Self Massage

Now that you have your Spa-Cipes oil, start to do massage trades with your partner or spouse.

I also highly recommend giving yourself lots of self massage. Here are just a couple of tips for effective ways to take care of yourself with self massage and some stretching.

Hand Massage

1. Take the thumb and forefinger of your right hand and press in the center of the left hand's web between the thumb and fore finger. Hold this for a few seconds. Start to move the thumb in a circular motion. Do a couple of circles.

2. Then, press with the thumb and fore finger each joint one by one. Do a press and then release 3 times, then go to another joint. Do all the fingers. Repeat other hand.

Wrist and Forearm Care

1. Rotate both of your wrists both directions. Do several rotations.

2. Make figure 8's in the air with both wrists. Do many of these.

3. Take both hands and turn the fingers towards you and place both hands down on a table, breathe into this stretch. Hold for 2 minutes. It can be intense, but keep breathing into it.

Neck Stretch and Massage

1. Rotate the neck slowly with your full range of motion several times both directions.

2. Using both hands place them at the base of the head and make small circles up and down to the neck.

3. Press your thumb into spots that are tender and take deep breaths, hold the spot and breathe into it.

4. Drop your head back and let it hang while you breathe and move the head from side to side. Think about letting go of the tension.

Shoulder Massage

1. Taking the opposite hand, grab the top of the opposite shoulder blade and pull out. feel for the tension and rub outward. Repeat other side.

2. With the same hand, make circles at the top of the shoulder.

3. Rotate shoulder back several times.

4. Drop the shoulders way down your back and focus on lifting the breast bone up with

shoulders down, and then hold that while breathing.

Lower Back Massage

1. Taking both hands, place them at your lower back, rubbing downward with your fingers using as much pressure as you can.

2. Turn the finger tips inward and pull the tissue away from the spine. Move as far up the back as you can reach.

3. Holding your hands on your lower back, lift the breast bone up and stretch back while breathing into the lower back.

Foot Massage

1. Sitting on the floor, in a chair or in a healing bath, bring your feet in so you can reach them. Using your hands, take a hold of both feet. Starting at the heel, rub your thumb up and down the arch of your foot, pressing on spots that are tender. This arch represents your spine, the heel being your lower back and under the big toe your shoulders. When you have issues in these areas, hold that spot and keep rubbing.

2. With your thumb on the top of the foot, starting at the ankle, draw a line with the thumb to each of the toes. Make small circles with your thumb on top of the foot.

Chapter Six
Hair Treatments

I used to brush my Mom's hair when I was a young girl. My Mom started to lose hair in her forties and she would tell me often that her hair was thinning and she worried about it. She started to wear wigs and hats. I remember being about 15 and seeing a hair regrowth food remedy treatment on a daytime talk show.

Somehow I talked my Mom into letting me do the experiment on her. This was the only time I was ever able to get her to be my client and she was not a very open one at that. But, she did sit through two of my treatments. I remember it was a crazy mixture with eggs, vinegar, beer and other herbs. She sat complaining that everything was cold. I did have fun cracking eggs onto her head, and then wrapping up her head and telling her to sit with it. Unhappily, she did as she was told. I do not think it worked well and I never got her to sit in my experiment chair again. Fortunately, I learned a great deal from my experiments.

Just recently, I have been focused on my own hair. I am going grey and with that comes frizzes and I want to keep healthy shining hair. A client told me to get Alma oil to get a thick and shining mane.

She told me that this oil is a Ayurvedic treatment and this is why Indian women have such dark, thick and beautifully shiny hair. I tried it, and wow! She was right! You can use this oil alone but, you know me, I love adding in food. I do just the oil massaged straight into my scalp at night so the oil can sit in my hair all night. Then, once a month, I do the Thick and Shiny Hair treatment and it solves my frizzy hair and brings back the deep shine in my hair. Not to mention, it's more manageable and lasts for weeks. I do the Alma oil in-between the Thick and Shiny Hair treatment about once or twice a week. I have been doing the Henna color every 3 weeks and it is making the grey look more like highlights, which looks really nice.

Thick and Shiny Hair

You will need a hair paint brush or comb
a shower cap
5 drops Alma oil
One blended avocado
1/2 cup water

Blend one avocado, add in water and Alma oil. Mix thoroughly. Apply to hair evenly and put on shower cap or wrap head in a towel to keep warm; let hair sit up to 20 minutes, rinse and dry. Take two drops of the Alma oil and rub it into your scalp again and let that sit all night. Wash your hair in the morning, and when you dry and style you will notice thick and shiny hair.

ENJOY!

Natural Hair Dye

Henna for Brown hair
You will need gloves, a bowl, strainer, hair cape or
towel, hair paint brush and/or a squeeze bottle.
1 cup henna brown or dark brown
1/2 cup boiling water
1 oz. shot apple cider vinegar

Add in boiling water to henna, stir, then add in used
coffee grounds (use leftovers from this morning's
coffee), and apple cider vinegar. Let mixture sit and
steep while it cools. Strain mixture into a new bowl or
squeeze bottle.
Apply mixture to hair using squeeze bottle or by
painting it on. Starting in the center of your head and
moving outward, make sure you cover all grey areas
and keep mixture away from skin on face as it may dye
it as well. Add coconut oil to the edge of your face to
avoid getting henna on your skin. Place shower cap or
plastic wrap over your head and let sit. You can sit
under a hair dryer or add heat for 45 to 60 mins. If you
do not want to sit with heat, leave your henna
treatment in for 60 – 75 mins. For more complete
coverage, leave in for up to 3 hours.

This is the color treatment I am now doing on my own hair to cover the grey. It works ok, but can be very messy. I have found it covers best when used about 4 weeks after a professional dye and then to continue to do it every 3 weeks for several months. Then you can start to spread out the dye times farther and farther away from each other. This color treatment will last 4 to 6 weeks and has no harsh chemicals.

Ok, so maybe you're not a brunette? You can still use Henna whatever color your hair is. Henna comes in many colors and adding in teas will give you just the color you'll Love.

Create your own colors! Purchase the Henna color of your choice: brown, dark brown, blonde or red, and then find which one below suits you and have fun playing with color.

- To tone down the reddish tint in the Henna, add in 1 cup used coffee grounds with your mixed Henna.
- For covering grey hair, add in 2 teaspoons apple cider vinegar. This helps the Henna stick to the grey hair.
- Lemon juice will lighten blonde shades. 2 tbsp juice to Henna mixture.
- Want some golden highlights? Mix in some teas: Ceylon or Black China Tea. Red Zinger Tea enriches red tones in the Burgundy, Sherry, Mahogany and Red Henna colors.
- Chamomile Tea brightens and adds a Neutral, Blonde, or Marigold Blonde Henna.

Let teas steep 20 -30 mins after bringing to boil.
Substitute tea for water, then mix as directed.

I was talking with a client recently about Henna
coloring and she brought us a trend that all the kids are
doing. They are using Koolaid to color hair and the
process as she explained it is a lot like the Henna
process. The Koolaid treatment will give hair the color
of the powder. I guess the kids are making streaks with
this powder by using foil and brushing on the color
they desire. This is not completely holistic but, I must
admit, Koolaid on the hair is better than in your body.
If you are looking for color streaks or all over colors on
your hair, try this instead of harsh coloring. It can last 4
to 6 weeks.

Egg on your face is good, but in your hair is just as
good. The yolk, rich in fats and proteins, is a natural
moisturizer. Egg whites contain bacteria-eating
enzymes that remove unwanted oils.

Egg Hair Treatments

You will need a bowl and hair paint brush
- For normal hair; use an entire egg or two
- For oily hair; use only the egg whites
- For dry brittle hair; use egg yolks only

Mix up to 1/2 cup of whichever egg mixture is appropriate for you and apply by painting on the mixture to clean, damp hair. If there isn't enough egg to coat scalp and hair, use more as needed. Leave on for 20 minutes, rinse with cool water (to prevent egg from "cooking") and shampoo hair. Whole egg and yolks-only treatments can be applied once a month; whites-only treatment can be applied every two weeks.

Does your hair seem dull? Are pollution and other hair products making your hair lifeless by leaving a film on your hair? The best treatment is located in your fridge. Dairy products like sour cream and yogurt may help reduce this damage. Lactic acid in the dairy strips away the build up and the milk fat moisturizes.

Dairy Hair Treatment

1/2 cup sour cream

Massage sour cream into damp hair and let sit for 20 minutes. Rinse with warm water, followed by cool water, then shampoo hair as you normally would. Treatment can be applied every other week.

Here is one more treatment to help rid your hair of buildup. Nothing eats through product build up like baking soda!

Baking Soda Buildup Reducer

1 to 2 Tbsp baking soda

water

Mix baking soda with small amounts of water until a thick paste forms. Massage into damp hair and let sit for 15 minutes. Rinse with water, then shampoo hair. Treatment can be applied every two weeks.

Got the frizzes? You already have the
Thick and Shiny treatment that I use.
You can also just use avocado to rid your hair of
the frizz. The oil in the avocado is what repairs the
damaged hair and gives you that soft shining hair.

Avocado Hair Treatment

1 avocado
1 to 2 Tbsp of sour cream
Mash up half an avocado and massage into clean,
damp hair. Let sit for 15 minutes before rinsing with
warm water. Treatment can be applied every two
weeks.

Too much oil has never been my problem but some of us do get oily scalp and hair. Soak up that oil by using corn starch and do some dry brushing to help remove excess oil and powder from the hair.

Oily Hair Treatment

You will need a shaker with holes in it
and a bristle hair brush
1 Tbsp. cornstarch

Pour powder into an empty shaker and sprinkle onto dry hair and scalp until you've used it all. After 10 minutes, use a natural bristle hairbrush to completely brush it out. Treatment can be applied every other day.

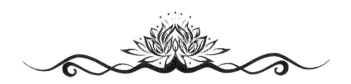

Itchy scalp is a problem that is no fun and can happen to dogs as well as in people. You can use the itchy scalp treatment on your dog as well. Let the treatment sit as long as the dog will let it sit. A lemon juice and olive oil mixture in your hair will rid your scalp of any loose, dry flakes of skin, while the olive oil moisturizes.

Itchy Scalp Treatment

You will need a bowl and a hair paint brush.
2 Tbsp fresh lemon juice
2 Tbsp olive oil
2 Tbsp water
Mix and massage into damp scalp. Let mixture sit for 20 minutes, then rinse and shampoo hair.
Treatment can be applied every other week.

Dry or Sun-Damaged Hair Treatment

You will need a bowl and a hair paint brush.
1/2 cup of honey
1 to 2 Tbsp olive oil
1 egg yoke
Mix ingredients and massage honey into clean, damp hair. Let sit for 20 minutes, then rinse with warm water.
Treatment can be applied once a month.

I'm not a beer drinker but we all have heard it is good to wash your hair in beer. Beer contains generous supplies of yeast, which works to plump tired hair.

Limp Hair Treatment

You will need container like a large glass
or a mason jar
1/2 cup flat beer
1 raw egg
I tsp avocado oil
Pour beer into a container and let it sit out for a couple of hours to deplete carbonation. Mix in egg and oil into a spray bottle. Spray on clean, damp hair, let sit for 15 minutes, then rinse with cool water. You can just use the beer in a spray bottle and spritz onto dry hair. When the liquid evaporates, the remaining protein residue continues to strengthen and structure hair. Store remaining in fridge and use every other day.

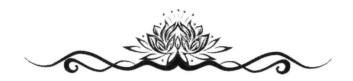

I have to admit I have never made a natural homemade shampoo. I did find a recipe that I will share here for you to try, using the wonder plant Jojoba. Native Americans used the salve to soften and heal skin and hair, along with preserving animal hides.

Jojoba Shampoo

You will need a bowl and a squeeze bottle.
1/4 cup coconut milk
1/3 cup liquid castile soap
1/2 of a teaspoon Jojoba oil
5 drops of Essential Oils
3 teaspoons avocado oil
Mix all of the ingredients into a bowl, being careful not to mix too much and create bubbles with the castile soap. Place mixture into the squeeze bottle.

I get asked a lot, "What can I do that's natural for hair loss?" The answer is my Fall favorite! Pumpkin is especially good for moisturizing dry or damaged hair and will help with re-growth of hair. Because of its rich source of potassium this makes pumpkin especially useful in promoting the re-growth of hair.

Pumpkin Hair Conditioner

2 cups pumpkin uncooked or canned (organic)
1 tablespoon coconut oil
1 tablespoon honey
1 tablespoon yogurt

In a food processor or blender, puree the pumpkin and yogurt. Add the coconut oil and honey after and ensure that the mixture is smooth. Apply to damp, shampooed hair. Cover with plastic cap and sit under the dryer for fifteen minutes. Rinse out thoroughly and style as usual. You can do this treatment weekly.

Now you can do those expensive hair treatments at home and when you are sitting in your hair treatment of choice, you can add one of the food facials. It is the best time to meditate, too. If you have my first book, you can look one up in there or go to Chapter Ten and do one of the Loving Your Body meditations. If you love to multi-task you will love multi-tasking while relaxing. If you meditate while doing your treatments, you will expand your healing 110%!

If you could see the energy you are creating, you would see a purple and white light beginning from within and expanding out several feet. You would see your heart opening and all the muscles in your body relaxing. You will notice deeper, more compete breathing and you may want to fall asleep. Give this time to yourself, not only to look prettier, but to stay in balance. When things feel out of my control, I do an at home spa treatment. When I am done, I may still be in the midst of chaos, but I do look and feel better.

Here is the secret to being able to pull off pampering yourself while feeling really crappy. I know this is what stops people from getting pampering, much less giving it to themselves. When you feel crappy, it is easy to want to grab a drink, vent to others, or just go to sleep. Withdrawing from things, not eating and then not taking care of yourself begins. Stop the negative pattern by scheduling your treatments on your calendar, then have them even if you have had a bad day or not feeling it. Do it anyway. This will start to begin that habit of being good to yourself.

What also makes it easier is to have all of your ingredients in your fridge. When at the store buying food, remember what you have tried here and always pick up some food for your face and hair. Having your bowls, brushes and other tools in a spot easily accessible helps because when you feel low, you will look for any excuse to get out of doing it. Thinking it is too much work is the biggest hurtle to get over. Now, your homework is to make a list of tools you need to get to do your face and hair treatments at home. Keep this list in your purse or a place where you will have it when you are out running errands. Get your items and then when you're home again, set up your spa drawer or cabinet in your bathroom and kitchen. You will be so happy you did this the next time you feel stressed!

Chapter Seven
Salt and Sugar Scrubs

We've talked about healing soaks, ways to hydrate the skin, hair, and face as well as detoxing them. Now, I want to give you some knowledge about exfoliation of the skin. Exfoliation is just as important as the hydration. When dead skin is not removed from the face, it will cause a buildup that can cause acne. Skin that is not exfoliated regularly can start to look dull and show tiny lines easily.

A quick salt or sugar scrub rubbed onto the face and body once a week will make all the difference in the world. Salt is a cleanser and not only will it cleanse the body of unwanted dead skin cells, it clears your energetic field of static energy and can start to move blocked energy. Do you ever wonder why going to the beach feels so good? After you go, you feel great! It's the salt water going to work and clearing your energy. Salt scrubs work in the same manner.

I like to use salt on my body and sugar on my face. I use coconut sugar but you can use any sugar you have. Your facial skin is delicate and sugar is a finer grain, and that is why I use it on the face versus using salt. The rest of the body can take a harder grain and deeper rubbing to really get in and clear the body and aura of blockages.

Whenever I start a body scrub, I start on the back and I always hear the clients say, "That feels great!" There is nothing like the feeling of getting your back scratched. Salt scrubs do this and more. It feels like a hundred hands are scratching your back. If you have a salt scrub with essential oils, the smells will give you the sense of being at the spa. I encourage couples to give each other back scrubs. If you're single, then I encourage you to get a professional body scrub so you can feel your back being scrubbed. Use the recipes in this chapter to give yourself scrubs in between having someone else give you one.

Foot scrubs are so wonderful when you have had a hard day. To get ready for a date or big day, do a scrub in the shower. There are lots of times to do scrubs and they are so easy to make. There is basically one easy way to make scrubs: 2 cups oil for every 1 cup of salt.

With the recipe being easy, it gives you many choices for what to add in as a scent and what type of oils to use. We will talk more about oils in the next chapter and there are many oils available to choose from.

Why Is Exfoliation Important?

The skin is constantly generating new skin cells at the lower layer (the dermis) and sending them to the surface (the epidermis). As the cells rise to the surface, they gradually die and become filled with keratin. These keratinized skin cells are essential because they give our skin its protective quality. But they are constantly sloughing off to make way for younger cells.

As we age, the process of cell turnover slows down. Cells start to pile up unevenly on the skin's surface, giving it a dry, rough, dull appearance. Exfoliation is beneficial because it removes those dead cells that are clinging on, revealing the fresher, younger skin cells below.

It is possible, however, to over exfoliate, especially on the delicate skin of the face. Over exfoliating will dry and irritate the skin. Set a schedule like once a week or every other week to do your exfoliation and you won't have the issue of over doing it.

Use the following recipes when you want to exfoliate skin. Add in essential oils to create your own type of treatment.

Basic Body Salt Scrub

You will need a bowl and spoon.
2 cups Epsom salts
1 cup oil of your choice
3 to 5 drops of essential oils of your choice
Mix using a spoon and store in cool dry place
or use right away.

Basic Facial Scrub

You will need a bowl and spoon.
2 tablespoons sugar (I like coconut sugar)
1 to 2 drops of essential oils of your choice
Mix using a spoon and store in cool dry place
or use right away.

Use when you have had a hard day on your feet
or if you have foot fungal issues or cracked heels.

Foot Salt Scrub

You will need a bowl and spoon.
2 cups Epsom salt
1 cup oil of your choice
3 to 5 tea tree oil
2 drops peppermint oil
1 drop rosemary oil
Mix using a spoon and store in cool dry place
or use right away.

Now that you know the easiest and most basic of
scrubs have fun with your newly found skill.
Salt Scrubs make great gifts!

Types of exfoliation

There are several types of exfoliation you can get at your local spa, but just two main types: the chemical type and mechanical type. You can go to the esthetician and get a peel to help problem skin and pay hundreds of dollars. These chemicals have enzymes, alpha-hydroxy acids (AHAs) or beta-hydroxy acids (BHAS) and they loosen the glue-like substance that holds the cells together, allowing them to slough away. Chemical peels can either be very gentle or very aggressive, depending on how the strong the peel is. The very aggressive peels will take off several layers of skin and leave you tender to the touch and pink faced. I recommend taking a gentler approach, try to not do anything aggressive at home.

We can create a gentle version of the chemical peel at home with food. When trying exfoliation for the first time, I suggest you try it on a small patch of the face or back of your hand. Make sure your skin is not going to have a reaction (a small percentage of people will have a reaction to food). Be mindful about how hard you are massaging in the scrub, starting off light and changing your pressure in areas that are dry, tender and more sensitive.

Use this scrub when you feel like you need a peel but want a gentler outcome.

Pineapple Scrub

You will need a bowl, a timer and two face cloths.
1 slice of pineapple
1 tablespoon pineapple juice
1 tablespoon oatmeal
1 tablespoon honey
2 drops of vitamin E oil

Mix all of the ingredients in a blender. Wet your face with warm water. Start massaging the scrub into your face and leave on for 5 minutes. You will feel a tingling, this is the enzymes in the pineapple working. Remove with cold wet cloth with vigorous upward strokes. End with a hydration of aloe lotion, coconut oil or a heavy night cream on your face. This treatment can be used once a month to help keep skin looking young and supple.

The Mechanical type of exfoliation is microdermabrasion. Microdermabrasion comes in two types - crystal and crystal-free, or diamond-tip and can be done by a professional or you can buy at-home replicas. I have had a couple of these treatments and I do feel I can create a comparably thorough exfoliation with the following Salt 'n Sugar facial scrub.

Use when you feel you need more of an exfoliation but can't get to the spa.

Salt 'n Sugar Scrub

You will need a bowl.
crystal salt
regular sugar
olive oil

Mix ingredients in the bowl. Gently rub in your mixture and wash off with warm water. Add an aloe lotion or light coconut oil to your face. This treatment can be used once a month to help keep skin looking young and supple.

Chapter Eight
Oils and Healing Steam

Over the years of being a massage therapist, I have learned a lot about oils. When I was growing up, we only had vegetable oil, mineral, and baby oil and that is all I knew. The varieties you can find now are amazing. The one I have most recently found is Coconut Oil. This gem of an oil has so many uses and benefits it is hard to list them all, but I will give you a good list. Start to use coconut oil for some of these things and you will notice a huge difference in the way your body feels and your skin looks. Coconut oil is a wonderful find, and there are many reasons why.

It's anti-inflammatory, antimicrobial, antifungal, antiviral, and improves nutrient absorption.

I was told put a spoonful of coconut oil in your coffee and it helps you from getting the jitters. When I want a second cup, I do this and it does work. How wonderful is that?

Beauty Uses

- Skin moisturizer – simply scoop some out of the jar and apply all over your body, including neck and face at night . The coconut oil is a bit greasy, so applying at night works best.

- Eye cream – apply under the eyes to reduce puffiness, bags, and wrinkles. Use on the lids in the evening. Using coconut oil around the eyes and on them will leave you a bit blurry eyed so again best to apply at night.

- As a skin preshave – coconut oil will prep skin for the pending damage caused by shaving.

- Aftershave – coconut oil will help heal your skin after shaving without clogging your pores.

- Deodorant – coconut oil alone can be used as a deodorant, but even more effective in combination with cornstarch and baking soda.

- Hair Conditioner/Deep Treatment – use as a leave in hair conditioner by applying a teaspoon of coconut oil to your ends and then running your fingers through your hair to distribute the rest! For a deeper treatment, follow the recipe in Chapter 5 for a deep conditioning treatment.

- Hair Gel/Defrizzer – rub a little between your palms and either scrunch into hair (for curly hair) or finger comb in through from scalp to ends (for wavy/straight hair).

- Toothpaste –mix coconut oil and baking soda and dab a little of the mix on your toothbrush.

- Make up remover – use a cotton swab and a dab of coconut oil and you'll be amazed at how well it works!

- Lip moisturizer – just rub a little into lips and it not only acts as a softening agent, but it also has an SPF of about 4 so you get a little protection!

- Massage Oil – pretty simple; grab some and rub! I use this a lot on clients with really dry skin.

- Lubricant – it is an all natural, perfectly safe personal lubricant. Not compatible with latex!

- Sunscreen – see Chapter Four for natural sunscreen recipe .

- Stretch Mark Cream – coconut oil is great at nourishing damaged skin. Mix with some vitamin E and you are well on your way to avoiding stretch marks during pregnancy.

- Nipple Cream – works great to nourish cracked, sore, or dry nipples. Apply to a cotton ball and leave on your nipples between feedings.

- Diaper salve – very comforting on a baby's bottom with no harsh chemicals.

- Cradle cap – having issues with dry skin on your baby's scalp? Coconut oil will not only nourish your baby's skin, it also helps eliminate cradle cap. Just rub a teaspoon onto scalp daily.

- Body scrub – add coconut oil to any of the recipes in Chapter Seven.

- Healing – when applied on scrapes and cuts, coconut oil forms a thin, chemical layer which protects the wound from outside dust, bacteria and viruses. Coconut oil speeds up the healing process of bruises by repairing damaged tissues.

- Bug Bites – when applied directly to a bug bite, coconut oil can stop the itching and burning sensation as well as hasten the healing process.

- Skin problems – coconut oil relieves skin problems such as psoriasis, dermatitis, and eczema.

- Swimmers Ear – mix garlic oil and coconut oil and put a few drops in the affected ear for about 10 minutes. Do this 2-3 times a day and it usually works within one or two days.

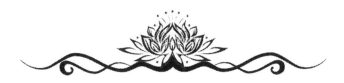

General Health and Wellness uses

- Stress Relief – relieve mental fatigue by applying coconut oil to the head in a circular, massaging motion. The natural aroma of coconuts is extremely soothing thus helping to lower your stress level.
- Digestion – when you ingest a couple table spoons; the saturated fats in coconut oil have anti-bacterial properties that help control parasites and fungi that cause indigestion and other digestion related problems, such as irritable bowel syndrome. The fat in coconut oil also aids in the absorption of vitamins, minerals and amino acids, making you healthier all around.
- Fitness – Also when ingested; coconut oil has been proven to stimulate your metabolism, improve thyroid function, and escalate energy

levels, all of which help decrease your unwanted fat, while increasing muscle.

- Nose bleeds – coconut oil can prevent nose bleeding that is caused by sensitivity to weather such as extreme heat and cold. This condition happens when the nasal passages become dry because of cold or dry air resulting in burns and cracks in the mucus membranes, causing bleeding. To prevent this, just put coconut oil in your nostrils. Coat your finger with coconut oil, and then lie down and insert your finger inside your nose. Doing this will strengthen and protect the capillaries in the nasal passages.

- For bleeding hemorrhoids, apply externally twice a day.

- Improvements in menstruation regarding pain/cramps and heavy blood flow

- May relieve acid reflux and indigestion when taken with each meal

- Cholesterol – improves HDL ('good' cholesterol) to LDL ('bad' cholesterol) ratio in people with high cholesterol

- Helps with canker sores, acne and cellulite.

- For herpes, apply topically and take internally.

- For genital warts, a thorough topical application over 6 weeks, and coconut oil enemas twice a day depending on the location of the warts.

Cooking

- Get more coconut oil in your diet! Use 1 cup to 1 cup ratio when replacing other oils/butter in recipes. A great replacement for various oils in liquid form – baking, cooking, sautéing, etc., and remember to add to your smoothies, too!

Other Uses

- Insect repellent – mix coconut oil with peppermint oil extract and rub it all over exposed skin.

- Great for dogs and cats for general wellness. Just add a teaspoon to their water bowl daily. They might just enjoy it straight, too!

- Goo Gone – just mix equal parts coconut oil and baking soda into a paste. Apply to the "sticky" area and let it set for a minute. Then, scrub off with an old toothbrush or the scrubby side of a sponge.

- Chewing Gum in Hair Remover – just rub some coconut oil over the stuck chewing gum, leave in for about 30 minutes, then roll the gum between your fingertips. Voila! It's out!

- Furniture Polish– coconut oil with a little bit of lemon juice to polish wood furniture. However, I recommend you test it first on a very small, unobtrusive part of your furniture to make sure it works the way you'd like.

- Polishing Bronze – all you have to do is rub a little oil into a cotton towel and then wipe down the statue. It cleans and helps deepen the color of your bronze.

- Seasoning animal hide drums.

- Seasoning cookware.

- Moisturizing and cleaning leather products.

Use this everyday to help with oral health, get glowing skin, and to help you stay well.

Oil Pulling

You will need a spoon.
Take a spoonful of coconut oil and swish in your mouth for up to 15 minutes.
When done, spit it out in the trash. Do not swallow the oil as it will transfer all the bacteria into your belly. Do not spit the coconut oil into the sink as it will clog your drain.

It's one of the easiest things you can do for your health! I oil pull while doing the dishes, feeding my animals, doing laundry, and vacuuming the house. I have been doing this for eight months and have seen many benefits including better dental check ups, not getting sick when I start to feel like I am and my neck and cheeks are getting a workout and are tightening up. It is like a face lift after weeks of oil pulling.

I have started to use hemp oil more, also. I am adding it in my smoothies and to my face scrubs. Hemp oil is a great non-clogging oil that helps to reduce the size of pores, blackheads, and acne. It also protects the skin from free radicals and provides the body with essential nutrients that help maintain the skin's water barrier, epidermal lipids, elasticity and softness. In addition, it has anti-inflammatory benefits, reduces redness and is recommended for the treatment of psoriasis and eczema. Omega-3s are particularly useful in reducing skin inflammation and redness.

There is information out there saying hemp oil is a great way to keep cancer away. If you have had a skin cancer removed, I recommend using the next recipe at least once a week, and adding hemp oil to your diet, also. One trick is to add hemp oil to your salads as a dressing.

Use this when your face needs a pick me up.

Hemp Oil Scrub

You will need a bowl and wash cloth.
1 tablespoon coconut sugar
2 tablespoons hemp oil
2 drops Vitamin E
With clean fingertips, rub and massage the mixture into your face, neck and if you like, the back of the hands and arms. Leave on to sit for up to 5 minutes. Use the wash cloth soaked in warm water to wipe off.

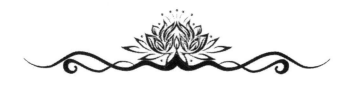

Steam

Steam has long been used as a therapeutic treatment. Eastern medicine has used steaming for centuries and other cultures have created spaces devoted to steaming for relaxation and detoxification.

Steaming can also be used as an excellent beauty treatment. Steam helps to balance complexions, clear away clogged pores, and lubricate skin. Steam helps in the treatment of acne, dehydration, and blackheads.

Estheticians often use the power of steam during facial services to soften the skin's surface and prepare it for pore extracting. However, steaming does not need to be performed by a professional; it can be done as a quick and simple treatment within the comfort of your home. Weekly steaming can be incorporated easily into your regular beauty routine to clarify the skin and promote a balanced complexion.

Use during or before you give yourself a facial or use alone as a mini facial.

Citrus Steam Facial

You will need a big bowl, bath towel,
and a way to heat water.
4 cups boiling water
2 drops of Blood Orange essential oil
1 drop of lemon oil or squeeze of real lemon
squeeze other citrus like pineapple or grapefruit

Add all the ingredients to the bowl and place the towel over your head, covering the bowl. Breathe in the steam deeply for as long as the water stays hot. Let the steam cover your face and neck. Wash face with gentle face wash after your steam. You'll feel so invigorated!

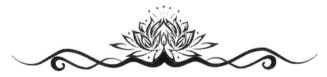

Use when you have a stubborn cough or congestion.

Steam Cough Remedy

You will need a big bowl, bath towel,
and a way to heat water.
4 cups boiling water
3 Pinches of parsley
3 drops of eucalyptus

Add all the ingredients to the bowl and place the towel
over your head, covering the bowl. Breathe in steam
deeply for as long as the water stays hot.
Do this up to 3 times a day to clear up cough and clear
breathing from colds and allergies.

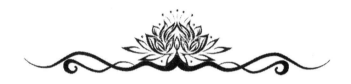

Use this as a stress reducer

and to help you sleep.

Lavender and Chamomile Steam

You will need a big bowl, bath towel and a way to heat
water.
4 cups boiling water
3 drops of lavender
4 drops chamomile
Add all the ingredients to the bowl and place the towel
over your head, covering the bowl. Breathe in steam
deeply for as long as the water stays hot.
Do this up to 3 times a day to clear up cough and clear
breathing from colds and allergies.

Chapter Nine
Feed Your Body

"If man makes it, don't eat it."

~Jack LaLanne

I met a lovely man this past year. All the work I have done on myself has finally brought me to the reason I was doing it all in the first place. I finally have found the love I was looking for.

The love is that of myself first, so that I can give and receive love in a healthy place. I am so grateful and glad I had enough courage to look deeply within, so I could be here now.

I am telling you this in this chapter because his showing up is significant with me changing my diet. All of these years, I have worked out and always had the belief that I could eat what I wanted because I am so active.

I was starting to feel sluggish and asked my new love to help me. He is a hypnotherapist and has great knowledge of food. He guides people to weight loss through his workshops, where he gives a lot of information about eating clean and through his hypnotherapy.

One hypnotherapy session and I was off sugar for a good several months. I remember taunting myself by standing in the ice cream section of the store, asking myself which one I wanted, and not wanting one at all! I would just walk away. During this time, we compiled a lot of information and created The Balance 7 Day Juice Cleanse. We use this cleanse to help our clients lose weight and we use it ourselves to keep cleansed and on track with our eating.

I am a fan of Balance, so Live Life! Eat dessert occasionally if you want when going out to dinner. Create healthy boundaries with your temptations, like having selected days of the week to indulge or only dark chocolate with fruit or nuts. Look for high end chocolates and learn how to bake a leaner cake for family birthdays. There are ways to have your cake and eat it, too. It is all just a conscious choice, like everything, right? Stay in the moment when you make your eating decisions. In this chapter, I will give you a lot of good information about achieving a good balance between your cleansing and eating.

Let the above quote sink in! I will repeat it again for you. Jack LaLanne, said, " If man makes it, don't eat it." We have all heard the horror stories of what is in our processed food, but still so many eat it! Why? Out of convenience?

I notice what excuses others use and the big one is many are convinced they do not have time to take care of themselves. I hear all the excuses, the beliefs and frankly, the "bulls**t"! As a community, we must teach and learn that there IS time to be healthy and there IS time to give to yourself. Just changing this belief will change your life. This new belief will give you the freedom you seek!

You are in charge of your thoughts and your schedule. Do not let excuses keep you stuck in the body you do not like, living a life you do not enjoy! Be in charge of yourself and take the time back. There is enough time when you start to believe there is. I would say that is the first step in making any changes in your life. Start with your thoughts, nothing will ever change when your thoughts are still telling you there is no time. Stop this battle inside your head because it is the only thing that keeps you stuck in conflict. Move out of conflict with yourself and into success!

There is a lot of data floating around about the food industry and all the bad things that are in our food. The words low fat, diet and healthy are placed on the product and we believe it! Why? Because we are stressed and have no time. Because we make these decisions in a not so present moment place. When you are in the present moment, you make the right decisions, always!

Doing this cleanse will give you enough tools that I guarantee you WILL want to continue to do it each and every day until it becomes a new way of life. New things will start to show up for you. Your life will become a wonderful adventure. Cleanses, whether it is of your home or body will start to move energy and any time you have movement of energy something needs to come in. It is a flow! Nature likes to flow. Just look at water: nature sets it up to flow in many different ways. Oceans and rivers flow, waterfalls flow, and little streams flow. When life flows in a balanced way, you feel ok with little stressors.

Waiting in line does not feel hard and stressful. Instead, you relax and enjoy the person in line with you or you're ok with being in the moment. I have made it my life's journey to find knowledge about how to do everything in balance. Life hands me situations to balance out all the time, just like it is handing it to you as well. I recognized this time during Spring 2013 to be the time I create a balance with my nutrition. As always, what information I gather, I document, and then send out into the world to help YOU. You will find a balance if you follow this guide and add to it what your intuition brings to you during the next 7 days.

Your journey is about to begin, so let me tell you a bit about what you will be doing.

The recipes in this chapter will awaken and rejuvenate your organs. If you happen to not do something in this cleanse, do not beat yourself up about it! Just start up again where you left off. No more beating yourself up, only loving yourself as you take on this journey. If you feel you may be critical of yourself, I suggest you take a couple of days before you start this program and follow the 2 day Loving Yourself guided meditations in Chapter Ten. While you are on The Balance 7 Day Juice Cleanse, do the Loving Yourself guided meditations daily.

Optimal health is a choice! Losing weight is a choice! Make the choice to experience life in a healthy way. Stop thinking about getting skinny or being on a diet. Think of it in terms of health and how you feel. It will take all of the stress off your mind about losing weight. Invest in things like a juicer or blender that can help you make veggie drinks. It is much easier to drink your veggies than to eat them. In order to get all the recommended amounts that we need to function at a high level of energy, we need to eat triple the amounts of fruits and vegetables we are eating. Many think this is too overwhelming, so instead choose the easy unhealthy road.

Maybe we do not know how to cook half of the good veggies we need and it just sounds like it all takes too much time. I know I felt this way and I was able to change it so I have the experience and soon you will, too. It is easier to stop at a fast food place to pick up dinner than to make it when you get home. I do get it! I was there myself. With this cleanse, however, you will not only have more energy, you will have more time because juicing is easier than cooking and easier on the cleanup of dishes. No more scraping off leftovers from meat on your pots and pans, at least for 7 days. I know juicers are harder to clean than the high speed blenders, so make your choice now of what you will want as you start this process.

I started with a juicer about five years ago. Juicers separated pulp from the juice and have some clean up involved. It takes a lot of veggies to get a small glass of juice. These types of juice drinks are meant to be an addition to your meals if you feel you already eat clean, but want more veggies in your diet. This may work better for you. There are lots of recipes where you can use the extra pulp so you don't waste it, baking the pulp into cakes, breads and soups. Cutting back on carbohydrates and meal portions while adding in fresh juices is a great way to start to get to know what veggies and fruit your body will respond to. Just getting more fresh veggies will give you more energy and is the best first step you can take.

This first step will lead into next steps like changing habits, shopping for clean food at stores and when eating out at restaurants. You will notice that you will start to skip whole aisles in the middle of the store and those aisles will start to really turn you off.

I had the privilege to gather most of this food information from Jack LaLanne himself. I asked him all about juicing and foods he allowed into his body, when I interviewed him in 2008. I learned a great deal in that hour, from this great Master of juicing. This cleanse is based mostly on that information.

I also need to credit a lot of this information to Dr. Oz, as he explained the three types of bodies and what foods helped those body types lose weight naturally. I have incorporated some of this information as a guide to help you with your body type. I am also explaining how some of the foods and herbs we will be using effect the body. With this information, using the recipes for cooking healthy meals while also doing some of the spa treatments (not necessarily all at the same time!), you will be feeling and looking fantastic in no time!

Since speaking with Jack LaLanne, I was juicing off and on. I would juice for a month or two as I still ate what I wanted. I was on the fence... questioning if I wanted to really make the change. Most of us sit in this place for a very long time, gaining weight! The place where we know what will give us optimal health and thus wealth but we do not really want to take the action to make it our reality. This past year, I started to feel sluggish a lot, especially in the afternoons. My clothes started to feel a bit tighter. I noticed a pain in my neck that massage was just not helping. Headaches started accruing more often due to congestion building on the left side of my face and head.

It really hit me when I had my yearly physical and my blood work came back low in Vitamins D and B. I had a scan done that scanned what level of antioxidants you have in your body and mine was very low. I am a healer and I was not at optimal health. I had to make a decision to change this or head down a path of becoming sick as I became older. This year was also a time that my Mother's health was going downhill fast. She broke a hip and was in and out of the hospital five times with life threatening situations. I could see myself at this place if I continued to eat the way I was.

Then, this documentary called Fat, Sick and Nearly Dead came into my life. It made me really think, I need to do this! I set out with my partner to create the Balance 7 Day Juice Cleanse, a cleanse that did not make me feel weak and sluggish. I wanted a meal replacement cleanse that would allow me to eat while juicing. One that could help me cleanse my organs; mostly liver and spleen. Also, clear my sinuses and maybe help me lose a couple of pounds. I started to think about Jack LaLanne's diet and all the other information I had gathered in the past five years. There had to be a balanced way to achieve my goal.

You can make this choice, like l did. I know this book can get you started onto the path of a balanced body. You will very soon love the body you are in if you just follow these instructions, I promise!!! How do I know you can do it? Because I have been there and I know your struggles! But I also know what it is like on the other side of it. I can help you cross that bridge that might scare you now.

From as far back as my great grandmother, the women in my family have struggled with weight, and I, too, have struggled with weight issues most of my life, Watching my mother's struggle when I was a young girl was heartbreaking, and it gave me the feeling of having a negative self image myself. I felt I had won the battle of the bulge in 2000, losing over sixty pounds. I have kept it off for over ten years. I had the mind set that I could lose weight just from exercising and doing my visualization work to overcome my negative body image. Working on these two parts of my life did help me to lose weight and keep it off, but it was just the beginning.

I made these changes while having the mind set that I could eat whatever I wanted because I worked out and I loved my body. I was not a veggie eating person back then, however, really only liking meat, pastas, potatoes and cake. Veggies had textures I did not like and they were cold. I did not know how to cook them to make them taste good. I had all kinds of excuses and reasons why not to eat them. I was healthy, I exercised daily and had changed my negative self image. I loved myself just as I was, there was no need to change my diet. It worked until I hit 45! My problem was not the weight now, it was how my organs were functioning. It was how tired I felt and how much pain I was feeling in my body as well as the positive encouragement that my boyfriend gave me that finally gave me the motivation to do it. I had been toying with this idea of doing a cleanse for too long. I decided that I had researched enough and my knowledge of what herbs and food to use to do a full body cleanse was good enough to start.

I purchased a Vita-Mix and got busy working on this cleanse. I decided if I was going to do this, I was going to do it right! I felt meal replacement was going to do it for me. I was pondering what other great teachers have taught me. When at a crossroads or when totally out of balance with a situation, go back to the beginning and start from there. Well, is that the same for eating?

I think so...juicing is going back to the beginning. Back to when we drank and ate smashed up baby food, then introducing solid foods slowly. We start off eating the right way and then somewhere along that journey we take the wrong road. This cleanse takes you back to the basics.

How To Begin?

1. Decide whether you would like to juice in a Juicer or make meals in a power blender. Purchase what you need if you do not have one already. Remember it is an investment in your health.
2. Decide when you want to begin. Put it on your calendar!
3. How long of a juice cleanse do you want to do? You can do as little as three days or keep it going for twenty one days.
4. Will you be doing the cleanse with anyone? Try to get your household on board with your cleanse, or maybe a co-worker or friend to keep each other accountable.
5. Clean out your kitchen. Throw away all temptations or put them on higher shelves.

6. Go shopping and get your healthy food. You will be surprised at the aisles in the store that you will completely avoid.

7. Be good to yourself! Give yourself love for the new life you are creating!

Shopping List

Vegetables

Tomatoes, carrots, spinach, kale, onion, green lettuces, celery

Red and green cabbage, broccoli, wheat grass, asparagus

Fruit

Lemons, pineapple, bananas, green grapes, red grapes, frozen strawberries, green apples, oranges, guava, frozen peaches, frozen or dried cranberry (be careful of the sugar in the dried fruit)

Herbs and Roots

Cilantro, parsley, cayenne pepper, Echinacea, hemp seed, turmeric, dandelion, caraway seed, comfrey, cinnamon, mint leaves, parsley

green tea

chamomile tea

ginger

beets

Nuts

almonds (preferably raw and unsalted)

walnuts (preferably raw and unsalted)

Oils and Vinegars
olive oil or grape seed oil is a healthier choice and can
be a substitution
coconut oil
apple cider vinegar
balsamic vinegar
Minerals
calcium bentonite clay
Juice
Aloe juice or water
Allowed Dairy
almond milk chocolate and vanilla
plain yogurt (the cleanest yogurt I could find is Fage
pronounced Fa-yeh)
Allowed Food
eggs (cage free or fresh if possible)
oatmeal (unsweetened)
Sugar Substitution
stevia
honey

"If more of us valued food and cheer
and song above hoarded gold,
it would be a merrier world."
– J.R.R. Tolkien

When making your smoothies, place all items into the blender or juicer and mix until smoothie texture. Most of the recipes make 2 to 3 quarts and will serve two or three. You may store extra in the refrigerator and drink it as a snack if you get hungry. If you want to make a recipe for one and do not want extra, simply cut recipe in half.

With the daily recipes you will be following, there are side dishes that are healthy choices for you to choose from if you feel like you cannot just juice and need some food. That is the beauty of doing something IN balance, it is not strict and one sided. There are always choices. If you are hungry, go to these food choices. They will be foods that taste good and that will nourish your body and keep the cleanse going . If you feel like you need sugar or something sweet in the middle of the day, by all means, make the night's dessert, saving half for after dinner. This cleanse is meant to be a balance, do not deprive yourself of anything. If you cave in and eat something not on the meal plan, do not beat yourself up and do not start over. There is no punishment here, only a continuation of the journey. If you are having difficulty with any of this cleanse, find support. It is best to get the support of family and friends before you begin and it is easier to do anything with a partner. If you need to, you may contact my office at melissa@balancestudio.org for any guidance you need.

Take advantage of doing the spa treatments. They will give you balance on the outside. Start to make time for yourself and you will notice just how much you really do love yourself and time with You.

On day 7, congratulate yourself and make a decision to how much of this cleanse you can keep in your life, and then keep going. Keep creating a balanced diet by following the recipes for day 8 until day 14. These are recipes that will include adding back in the foods we were not eating, slowly and gradually.

After day 14, you deserve a great deal of respect and will feel so proud. You will have enough knowledge to continue on and make your own food choices. Come back to this book when you feel like balance needs to be attained. Have fun with these recipes and make up some of your own. Once you learn what herbs to use for what and what veggies help which organs, you can become a manager of your own health. Make day 15 to 21 your own creations to capture the health and well being you want to see in your life. Find what is best for your body type and palate and play with it. Create art with your eating and it will serve you in a healthy and wealthy way.

Which body type you are tells you a story, says Dr. Oz:

Apple-shaped body type

Apple-shaped women tend to hold excess body fat in their waists, arms and breasts with very little body fat stored in their lower bodies. Apple-shaped bodies should eat foods low on the glycemic index. Reducing or eliminating carbs from an Apple's diet prevents a spike in blood sugar and keeps cortisol controlled. The less cortisol, the less belly fat.

Apple body types can replace simple carbs with the following foods:

- Lentils, which are packed with protein and require more energy for the body to break down.

- Red pepper hummus, also rich in protein; the spices can also boost metabolism.

- Eggplant makes a great carb substitute. When used in certain recipes, for example an eggplant lasagna, it gives you the same density and texture as pasta.

Pear-shaped body type

Pear-shaped women, on the other hand, tend to carry extra pounds in their lower bodies, rather than gaining in the waist or upper body. Pears are plagued by what many of you may know as "junk in the trunk." Pears carry most of their weight on their lower hips, thighs and butt. And perhaps most frustrating of all, a stubborn pooch of tummy fat. While it may take longer to accumulate this kind of fat, it's also much harder to get rid of. Why? This kind of fat is influenced by estrogen, and estrogen helps make fat. When a woman gets pregnant, estrogen spikes (which is why many women keep the weight on long after the baby is born). When a woman has a heavy period, estrogen spikes – making more fat. The good news is, this kind of fat is not as dangerous as belly fat, but it may be more unsightly, as it can become that cheesy, cellulite-type fat that is every woman's nightmare. And while an Apple cannot become a Pear, with excessive weight gain, a Pear may wind up transforming into an Apple.

Pears are at a higher risk for osteoporosis. During menopause, Pears make much weaker estrogen, which is not strong enough to keep calcium in the bones. Other health issues for this type are cellulite, varicose veins and joint problems.

The secret: high-fiber foods. Fiber binds to the estrogen in your gut and carries it out of your body when you go to the bathroom. Keeping your body's estrogen in balance in this manner can enhance your weight-loss efforts and improve your silhouette.

Pears can try these high-fiber foods:

- Edamame, rich in phytoestrogens to regulate your estrogen levels.

- Whole-wheat pasta – a great swap for regular pasta that will fill you up fast.

- Figs are a fruit with one of the highest levels of fiber. If you have a sweet tooth, dried figs are a healthy way to help you get your fix.

Boxy body type

If you find yourself possessing the attributes of both an Apple and a Pear, you are likely a Box body type. Unfortunately, as America's weight problem continues to grow, this body type is also on the rise. This body type is most concerning because of its wide range of health implications: It affects the thyroid gland, and those carrying excess weight with this body type can run a greater risk of experiencing depression, memory loss, high cholesterol and an enlarged heart.

If you are a Box and you are lacking enough thyroid hormones, every cell in the body gets fatter due to a slowing of your overall metabolism. Since the thyroid controls the metabolism, all the body processes are slowed, including digestion, mental clarity, and even absorption of vitamins.

The Box shape is regulated by the thyroid hormone. A healthy thyroid speeds up the metabolism.

The secret for Boxes to turbocharge their metabolism: Foods high in selenium and iodine. Iodine is vital for healthy thyroid hormone production, and the essential mineral selenium may help decrease inflammation that can cause an underactive thyroid. Today, many people use kosher salt or sea salt, but these salts do not contain iodine. To help maintain healthy thyroid function, reach for traditional iodized table salt when seasoning food.

You can also try the following foods:

- Seaweed, a great snack packed with both nutrients and iodine.

- Shrimp - it's also a good source of vitamin D

- Sunflower seeds, just one-third of a cup makes for a great daily snack

Use the body type guide with your cleanse. For example, I am a pear shape and I add figs into my smoothies. Feel free to add in any of the foods that are explained in the following lists.

Why we are using these herbs, oils and minerals in the Balance 7 Day Juice Cleanse?

Herbs and Roots

Cilantro protects against Salmonella, is a good source of fiber, helps bind to heavy metals in your body, is a great anti-inflammatory herb, rich in magnesium, iron and phytonutrients, lowers blood sugar, relieves intestinal gas, and prevents nausea.

Parsley is rich in many vital vitamins, including Vitamin C, B 12, K and A. This means parsley keeps your immune system strong, tones your bones and heals the nervous system. It helps flush out excess fluid from the body, thus supporting kidney function. However, the herb contains oxalates, which can cause problems for those with existing kidney and gall bladder problems. Please omit this herb if you have these problems. The herb has anti-inflammatory properties and relaxes stiff muscles and encourages digestion.

Cayenne pepper has anti-irritant properties, is an anti cold and flu agent, digestive aid, anti-fungal, anti allergen, anti bacterial, a joint pain reliever and can help keep headaches away.

Echinacea helps build a strong immunity and can keep colds and flu away.

Hemp Seeds one of the most potent foods available as they support optimal health and well being. Hemp seeds aid in weight loss, increased and sustained energy, rapid recovery from disease or injury, lowered cholesterol and blood pressure, reduced inflammation, improvement in circulation and immune system as well as natural blood sugar control.

Turmeric is a natural liver detoxifier, and has long been used in Chinese medicine as a treatment for depression. It is a potent natural anti-inflammatory that works as well as many anti-inflammatory drugs but without the side effects. May aid in fat metabolism and help in weight management.

Dandelion is a digestive aid, liver and kidney detox, acts against cancer and is rich with antioxidants.

Caraway Seeds are a rich source of dietary fiber. The seeds are a storehouse for many vital vitamins. Vitamin A, Vitamin E, Vitamin C as well as many B-complex vitamins like thiamine, pyridoxine, riboflavin, and niacin particularly are concentrated in the caraway seeds.

Cinnamon may lower blood sugar in people with type 1 or type 2 diabetes, according to Diabetes UK. A chemical found in Cassia cinnamon - can help fight against bacterial and fungal infections.

Mint Leaves are soothing to the digestive tract, reduces irritable bowel syndrome, cleanses the stomach and also clears up skin disorders such as acne. Mint helps in eliminating toxins from the body. Mint is a very good cleanser for the blood.

Green Tea helps burns fat to aid in weight loss.

Chamomile tea helps to calm the body and promote sleep.

Ginger helps with digestion.

Beets are a high source of energy and helps cleanse the liver. High in potassium, magnesium, fiber, phosphorus, iron; vitamins A, B & C; beta-carotene, beta-cyanine; folic acid.

Clay

Calcium Bentonite Clay is highly charged with negative ions. Dry calcium bentonite clay is inert. It attracts positive ions when 'activated' through hydration. Once hydrated, the negative ions are 'living' and begin their work of attracting free radicals, impurities and other toxins. The clay is not absorbed by the body, but does its job as it passes through and is then eliminated.

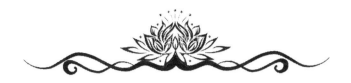

Why we are using these foods in the Balance 7 Day Juice Cleanse?

Vegetables

Asparagus contains vitamin A for better vision, potassium for smooth kidney functioning, and trace minerals that help boost immunity. Asparagus is a rich source of B vitamins, which are known to regulate blood sugar levels.

Broccoli has a strong, positive impact on our body's detoxification system.

Carrots increase saliva and supply essential minerals, vitamins and enzymes that aid in the digestion process. They are rich in alkaline elements, which purify and revitalize the blood while balancing the acid/alkaline ratio of the body.

Celery reduces inflammation, it regulates the body's alkaline balance and aids in digestion.

Green lettuces contains Vitamin A, Vitamin C and Vitamin K.

Kale is high in fiber, high in iron, Vitamin A, Vitamin C and calcium. Kale is a great detox food and is an anti inflammatory. Great for cardiovascular support.

Onion contains chromium, which assists in regulating blood sugar.

Red and Green Cabbage Vitamin A, Vitamin C, Vitamin K and Iron.

Spinach very good for digestion and it also flushes out toxins from the colon.

Tomatoes are high in Vitamin A, Vitamin C, Calcium and Potassium. They are the best food sources of lycopene according to the Tomato Research Council in New York City. They help your skin, eyes and can protect against heart disease. We are using tomatoes to help support heart function and to help your skin and eyes.

Wheat Grass is a energy booster and it contains Chlorophyll. Chlorophyll is antibacterial and can be used inside and outside the body as a natural healer. Chlorophyll neutralizes toxins in the body.

Fruit

Lemons are acidic to the taste, but are alkaline-forming in the body. In fact they are one of the most alkaline-forming foods; this makes them great for balancing a highly acidic condition in the body. They are rich in vitamin C that works against infections like the flu and colds.

Bananas can reduce swelling, protect against type 2 diabetes, aid weight loss, strengthen the nervous system, and help with the production of white blood cells, all due to high levels of vitamin B-6.

Green Grapes One cup of grapes, with about 100 calories, provides more than a quarter of the daily recommended values of vitamins K and C. Grape seeds, which are edible, are chock-full of antioxidants.

Red Grapes have a property called resveratrol and this property aids in weight loss and is anti-inflammatory.

Strawberry's red coloring contain anthocyanins, which stimulate the burning of stored fat. Strawberries contain potassium, vitamin K and magnesium which are important for bone health

Apples help to control your weight, detoxify your liver and boost your immune system.

Oranges have polyphenols and can protect against viral infections. Oranges give you energy and are packed full of full of beta-carotene, which is a powerful antioxidant.

Guava can aid in weight loss and thyroid health.
Peaches have a diuretic effect which helps cleanse your kidneys and bladder and can aid in weight loss.

Cranberry aids in bladder and gastrointestinal health.

Pineapples have exceptional juiciness and a vibrant tropical flavor that balances the tastes of sweet and tart. Pineapples can help boost metabolism and aid in weight loss. They are second only to bananas as America's favorite tropical fruit.

Nuts

Almonds and **Walnuts** for protein and to feel full. Almonds are high in monounsaturated fats, the same type of health-promoting fats as are found in olive oil.

Juice/Milk

Aloe Juice Aloe Vera contains many vitamins including A, C, E, folic acid, choline, B1, B2, B3 (niacin), B6. Aloe Vera is also one of the few plants that contain vitamin B12.

Some of the 20 minerals found in Aloe Vera include: calcium, magnesium, zinc, chromium, selenium, sodium, iron, potassium, copper, and manganese.

Almond Milk In unsweetened, chocolate and vanilla, a great substitute for cow and soy milk, with only 1/2 to 1/4 the sugars of cow's milk!

Allowed Whole Food
Eggs for protein and to help you feel full.
Oatmeal for fiber benefits and to feel full.

Sugar Substitution
Stevia Sweet, but has no effect on blood sugars
Honey Natural sweetener with antibiotic properties

Day 1

Breakfast
2 glasses of water
Green Smoothie
1 Banana
Tea or coffee (you may keep coffee in this cleanse,
switch to decaffeinated if you like)

Green Smoothie recipe
1 1/2 cups water
1 head washed romaine lettuce
1 apple, cut up
1 pear, cut up
1 banana, peeled
1 lemon, peeled and seeded
1/3 bunch parsley
Pinch of echinacea
Pinch of dandelion
1 tablespoon calcium bentonite clay

AM Snack
1 glass of water
Wheat Grass shot
left over smoothie
apple

Wheat Grass recipe
1/3 cut wheat grass
1/2 cup water
strain into glass from blender or juice glass

Lunch
2 glasses of water
Detox Smoothie

Detox Smoothie recipe
1 1/2 cups water
1/2 lemon, peeled and seeded
1 pear, cut up
1 green apple, cut up
1 tablespoon coconut oil
1/4 teaspoon turmeric
1/2 tablespoon ginger root
Pinch of cayenne pepper
Pinch of echinacea
Pinch of dandelion
1 tablespoon calcium bentonite clay
1/2 teaspoon stevia

PM snack
1 glass of water
1 orange
Green tea

Dinner
2 glasses of water
Cabbage Peach and Carrot Smoothie
Kale and Red Cabbage Salad with Olive Oil and Lemon
Juice dressing
Berry Blast Dessert

Cabbage Peach and Carrot Smoothie recipe
1/2 water
3/4 cup green cabbage
1 cup red grapes
1 carrot
1 cup frozen peach slices
1/2 cup ice cubes
Pinch of echinacea
Pinch of dandelion
1 tablespoon calcium bentonite clay

Kale and Red Cabbage Salad recipe
1 to 2 cups kale
1 cup chopped red cabbage
2 tablespoons olive oil
(oil massaged into kale gives better digestion results)
2 hard boiled eggs
squeezed lemon to taste

side suggestions if you feel hungry
steamed broccoli

Berry Blast Dessert recipe
2 frozen bananas
1 1/2 cup vanilla almond milk
1 cup frozen strawberrys
1 cup frozen blueberries

"One cannot think well, love well, sleep well,
if one has not dined well."
~ Virginia Woolf

Day 2

Breakfast
2 glasses of water
Banana Split Power Smoothie
2 hard boiled eggs or a scramble with spinach leaves
tea or coffee

Banana Split Power Smoothie recipe
1 cup vanilla almond milk
1 cup plain yogurt
1/2 banana, peeled
1 cup frozen strawberries
1 1/2 cup pineapple, chunks
1/2 teaspoon stevia
1 teaspoon clay

AM snack
1 glass water
wheat grass shot
1 cup red grapes
1 handful almonds

Lunch
2 glasses of lemon water
everything smoothie
small spinach salad with balsamic and apple cider
vinegar

Everything Smoothie recipe
1/2 cup vanilla almond milk
1/2 cup red grapes
1 peeled orange
1/2 pineapple - in chunks
1/2 small carrot
1/2 cup broccoli
1/2 cup spinach
1/2 cup frozen peaches
1 cup strawberries
1/4 banana peeled frozen
1 teaspoon clay

Spinach Salad recipe
1 to 2 cups uncooked spinach leaves
1 tomato, cut up
1 tablespoon balsamic vinegar
1 teaspoon apple cider vinegar

PM snack
1 glass water
1 shot or 2 tablespoons apple cider vinegar
1 apple

Dinner
2 glasses of water
Detoxifying Drink
Green Leaf Salad
Chamomile tea
Chocolate Pudding

Detox Drink recipe
2 cups green grapes
1 cup parsley
1 cup water or ice cubes

Green Salad recipe
1 to 2 cups green lettuce
1 cup red cabbage
1 to 2 tomatoes, sliced
1/2 cucumber, sliced

Chocolate Pudding recipe
1 avocado
1 tablespoon unsweetened chocolate powder
1/2 teaspoon honey to taste

Side suggestion if you feel hungry
Baked sweet potato

Day 3

Breakfast
2 glasses of water
Banana Apple Oatmeal Smoothie
slice of pineapple
tea or coffee

Banana Apple Oatmeal Smoothie recipe
1 cup water
1/4 cup plain yogurt
1/2 peeled banana
2 tablespoons uncooked oats
1/2 apple
1/4 cup dried cranberries
1/8 teaspoon ground cinnamon
1 teaspoon clay

AM snack
Wheat grass shot
Pear

Lunch
2 glasses of water with lemon
Detox Drink
Spinach Salad with hard boiled eggs
Cauliflower Mash

Detox Drink recipe
2 cups green grapes
1 cup parsley
1 cup water or ice cubes

Spinach Salad recipe

Cauliflower Mash recipe
1 head of cauliflower, cooked
2 small sweet potatoes, cooked
1 cup almond milk

PM snack
handful of almonds
green tea

Dinner
2 glasses of water
Cabbage Soup
Green Salad

Cabbage Soup recipe
2 cups veggie broth
1/2 cup chopped onion
1/2 carrot
1 sweet potato
1/4 teaspoon caraway seed
1 teaspoon dried dill weed

1/4 hot sauce
a Pinch of salt
Pinch of black pepper
4 cups cabbage

Green Salad recipe
green lettuce
tomatoes
cucumber

"I am a better person
when I have less on my plate."
~ Elizabeth Gilbert, Eat, Pray, Love

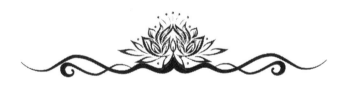

Day 4

<u>Breakfast</u>
2 glasses of water
Triple Berry Smoothie
apple
tea or coffee

Triple Berry Smoothie recipe
1/4 cup water
1/4 plain yogurt
1/2 cup strawberries
1/2 cup frozen blueberries
1/2 cup frozen raspberries
1 teaspoon clay

AM snack
1 glass water
Detox Drink
An orange

Detox Drink recipe
2 cups green grapes
1 cup parsley
1 cup water or ice cubes

Lunch
2 glasses of water
Green Smoothie

Green Smoothie recipe
1 1/2 cups water
1 head romaine lettuce
1/2 bunch spinach
1 apple
1 pear
1 banana
1 peeled and seeded lemon
1/3 bunch parsley
1 teaspoon clay

PM snack
1 glass water
Wheat Grass shot

Dinner
2 glasses of water
Nutty Fruit Smoothie
Strawberry Freeze

Nutty Fruit Smoothie recipe
1/2 cup water
1/3 cup plain yogurt
1/4 banana
2 tablespoons walnuts
1 tablespoon almonds
1 tablespoon honey
1/2 cup frozen raspberries
1 cup ice cubes

Strawberry Freeze recipe
2 frozen bananas
1 1/2 cup vanilla almond milk
1 cup frozen strawberry
2 figs

Day 5

Breakfast
2 glasses of water
Detox Smoothie
tea or coffee

Detox Smoothie recipe
1 1/2 water
1/2 lemon peeled and seeded
1 pear
1 green apple
1 tablespoon coconut oil
1/4 teaspoon turmeric
1/2 tablespoon ginger root
Pinch of cayenne pepper
1/2 teaspoon stevia

AM Snack
1 glass water
wheat grass shot
apple

Lunch
2 glasses water
Everything Smoothie

Everything Smoothie recipe
1 1/2 cups water
1 head romaine lettuce
1/2 bunch spinach
1 apple, sliced
1 pear, sliced
1 banana, peeled
1 lemon, peeled and seeded
1/3 bunch parsley

PM snack
1 glass of water
Apple Juice with Aloe Drink

Apple Juice with Aloe Drink recipe
4 apples
1/2 cup of aloe water or juice

Dinner
2 glasses of water
Cream of Asparagus Soup
Carrot Smoothie
Chocolate Banana Malt
Ginger Root and Mint Leaf tea
Cream of Asparagus Soup recipe
1/1/2 pounds cooked asparagus
1/1/2 cups veggie broth
1/2 cup vanilla almond milk

Carrot Smoothie recipe
1/2 cup water
1 cup red grapes
1 carrots
1 cup frozen peaches
1/2 cup ice cubes
Pinch of turmeric
1 tablespoon calcium bentonite clay

Ginger Root and Mint Leaf Tea recipe
1 teaspoon ginger root
2 leaves mint
1 cup hot water

Chocolate Banana Malt recipe
1 cup vanilla yogurt
1/1/2 vanilla almond milk
1/3 cup unsweetened choc powder
1/2 frozen banana
1 cup ice cubes

"All you need is love. But a little chocolate
now and then doesn't hurt."
— Charles M. Schulz

Day 6

Breakfast
2 glasses of water
Sweet Greens Smoothie
cooked whole oatmeal with sliced
apple and cinnamon to taste
tea or coffee

Sweet Greens Smoothie recipe
1/3 cup of water
1/2 cup chopped cucumber
1 cup spinach
1 cup frozen strawberries

Am snack
1 cup water
Detox Drink
Orange

Detox Drink recipe
1 cup green grapes
1 bunch parsley
1 cup water or ice cubes

Lunch
2 glasses water with lemon
Tomato Kale Smoothie
Spinach Salad
green tea

Tomato Kale Detox Smoothie recipe
3 Tomatoes
2 cups Kale
1 clove garlic
1 Pinch cayenne pepper
1 Pinch turmeric

Spinach Salad recipe
1 to 2 cups uncooked spinach leaves
1 cup grated carrot
1 tomato, chopped
1/2 cup peas
3 hard boiled eggs, sliced

Apple Cider Dressing recipe
2 tablespoons apple cider vinegar
1 tablespoon balsamic vinegar
3 tablespoons olive oil
1 clove garlic
2 large pinches of ground pepper
1 large pinch of sea salt
1 pinch turmeric
1 teaspoon honey to taste

PM Snack
1 glass water
wheat grass shot
apple

Dinner
2 glasses water
Tomato Soup
Tropical Energy Drink
Pineapple Ice Cream
Chamomile tea

Tomato Soup recipe
1 cup plain yogurt
3 tomatoes
1 tablespoon chopped onion
1/4 teaspoon dill weed
Sea salt

Tropical Energy Drink recipe
1 cup chopped pineapple
1 cup guava
1 cup aloe water
2 teaspoons coconut oil
honey to taste

Pineapple Ice Cream recipe
1 cup chopped pineapple
1/2 cup vanilla almond milk
coconut oil

Day 7

Breakfast
2 glasses of water
Peachy Green Smoothie
Scrambled eggs with uncooked spinach leaves
Tea or coffee

Peachy Green Smoothie recipe
1 cup vanilla almond milk
2 cups uncooked spinach
1 green apple, sliced
2 cups frozen peaches

AM Snack
1 glass of water
Detox Drink
orange

Detox Drink recipe
1 cup green grapes
1 bunch parsley
1 cup water or ice cubes

Lunch
2 glasses of water
Going Green Smoothie
Kale and Red Salad with Balsamic Dressing

Going Green Smoothie recipe
1/2 cup water
1 cup green grapes
1/2 fresh pineapple, cut up
1/2 banana, peeled
2 cups uncooked spinach
1/2 cup ice cubes
1 tablespoon calcium bentonite clay
Pinch of dandelion

Kale and Red Salad recipe
1 to 2 cups kale
1 cup chopped red cabbage
2 tablespoons olive oil
(oil massaged into kale gives better digestion results)
2 hard boiled eggs
squeezed lemon to taste

PM Snack
1 glass of water
shot of wheat grass
handful of walnuts
handful of red grapes

Dinner
2 glasses of water
Going Green Smoothie with Broccoli
Sweet Potato mash
steamed broccoli

Chapter Ten
Loving Your Body

The center of everything is the core of our bodies. It is the center of our being. This is where the solar plexus chakra (energy center) is located and all of our potential power is held. Also, the sacral chakra where we store emotional well being and this chakra is tied to our diet and exercise. I will go into chakras very little in this book. If you want more simple information about them, my first book will help you with this energy body knowledge.

The media and societies emphasis is on telling us we need to hide our bellies unless we have six pack abs. Hollywood portrays women as beautiful if they have no belly or shapely curves.

As voluptuous Goddesses we know better! Women that have well rounded bellies and lots of curves are true Goddesses. Our bellies are real, beautiful and make us the Goddesses we are. We come in all shapes and sizes and there is nothing wrong with any of us. It is only a mind set. Mind sets can be changed.

When starting to change your mind it may be difficult to let go of sucking in the belly, hiding it, and releasing this deeply seeded mind set. Self-esteem and confidence may be suffering because of old emotions surrounding your belly and negative body image. When the goal is to be a certain way, your potential power and journey is lost. You are not living in present moment but instead looking into the future.

Wishing your body to be different can affect your decision making and you care less about taking care of you. You can start to lose confidence in your own abilities.

Reclaim your femininity and beauty by putting you first and doing a lot of the suggestions in this book. It is a blessing to have a voluptuous body, one of a Goddess. I have a shapely figure, with strong muscles, bigger hips, a belly and a healthy sized chest. In reality, I never look good skinny. I once starved myself down to a size 5. I remember a friends dad told me I looked sick. He was right and his comment did make me think. I have since changed my mind set to being healthy instead of being skinny. Whatever healthy looked like for my body is ok with me, as long as I stay strong, flexible and healthy. I now know that I am a healthy Groovy Goddess! This is my body and the way it is supposed to look and it is fine with me.

"Change the way you look at things and the things you look at change."
— Wayne W. Dyer

A healthy body has nothing to do with your shape nor your size. We are all individuals and need be proud of the body we have to have well-being and peace in our hearts. To be happy in your own skin and love every inch of you will bring you the healthiest body each day.

Start today to love your body right now, this very minute as you read this. Love it for being able to carry you through your journey and being able to create your wonderful life.

To change how you see how you look, try using my Mirror, Mirror - Body Visualization. If you do not have a full size mirror, get one now! I started doing this not really understanding what I was doing. Along with changing my mind set, I lost weight and my body became more toned as I enjoyed my journey. Next time you get out of the shower, try this.

Mirror, Mirror - Body Visualization

Find your full length mirror and stand naked in front of it. Take a good look at your body. If negative thoughts come up, say " I love this body". Look at what you would like to change, start with one thing. Pull the skin tight to see what you would like to see and see it! Stare at it imprinting it in your mind, feeling as if you are this way already. Do this every day to all the parts of the body you would like to see change. Then, release it and go about your day loving the body you are in.

Along with using the visualization you can do abdominal exercises that strengthen your core. Building strong and flexible core muscles will help your posture. You look better when you hold your posture correctly.

The abdominals are made up of six muscles that all affect your posture and help in maintaining a healthy spine.

- The deepest of the muscle group is the **transverse abdominal muscles.** These muscles help in stabilizing your back and have a tremendous effect on body posture. As it wraps around the torso, creating an effect similar to a back support belt.
- The **internal obliques** are a pair of muscles, residing on each side of the torso. They are the next deepest, after the transversus. They also affect body posture. The internal obliques are involved in, among other things, rotation and lateral flexion of the spine.
- The **external obliques** are another pair of muscles that are located on either side of the torso, the love handles. Like the internal obliques, the external obliques are involved in, among other things, rotation and lateral flexion of the spine.
- The **rectus abdominus muscle** is the most superficial of the abdominal muscles. It and the external obliques affect body posture, just not as much as the deeper internal obliques and transversus muscles.

These are all the muscles that work in groups called the abdominal muscles. They are the spinal flexors. Their main job is to bend the spine forward, when contracting concentrically. The back muscles counterbalance the action of the abs, and are called spinal extensors. When the abdominals shorten to flex the spine, the back muscles are put on a stretch, and vice versa.

The abdominals also help in us participate in breathing especially during exhale, when they help force air out of the lungs by depressing the thorax.

I love to use an exercise ball to help in strengthening my ab muscles. Just sitting on the ball helps to contract through the abdominals. Make sure your ball is the correct height for you, and the package will give you guidelines on this. As you sit on the ball, your thighs should be level. The advantages to using an exercise ball is that it penetrates all of your core muscles and adds resistance. The ball gives you more angles of effort and helps to work through a full range of motion on multiple levels. Plus, it's fun!

Abdominal Curls

Movement One
Lie on your back with the ball under your knees, keeping the knees inline with the hips.
Hands placed behind the head or across your chest.
Inhale, prepare to lift, then exhale pulling the navel into the spine as you lift the upper body up, hold, then return your upper body to the mat. Repeat 8 to 10 times, slow and controlled.

Movement Two
Begin in the same starting position. Inhale, prepare to lift, then exhale a count of three as you lift the upper body up, making each movement its own count and breath. Repeat 8 to 10 times, slow and controlled.

Movement Three
Pick the ball up in your feet, lift it in the air, and place it in your hands. Feet flat on the floor with knees bent. Set the ball on your rib cage, hands at the side of the ball. Inhale, prepare to lift, then exhale, pulling the navel into the spine. Roll the ball up to your legs as you lift the head and shoulders. Inhale, hold this position, then exhale and return the head to the floor.
Repeat 8 to 10 times, slow and controlled.

Movement Four

Sitting on the ball, feet flat, knees bent, do a backbend on the ball to prepare and stretch. Hands behind the head or across the chest, inhale, prepare to lift, and then exhale, lifting the upper body up and crunch. Hold, then roll back down to the ball. Repeat 8 to 10 times, slow and controlled.

Movement Five

Still sitting on the ball, begin in the same starting position. Inhale, prepare to lift, exhale a count of three as you lift the upper body up, making each movement its own count and breath. Repeat 8 to 10 times, slowly and controlled.

Playing Throw and Catch

Back to the floor, place the ball between your feet and throw the ball to your hands.
Play catch back and forth and have fun. Repeat as many times as you want.

"Find your strength and love for your belly as you remember the playfulness of youth."

~ The Groovy Goddess

Oprah Winfrey's been on the path of Balance for some time. Funny story, I had a call one night from a neighbor. She had recorded an episode of Oprah when it was still on in the afternoon. She told me to come over to watch it, saying that I would not believe it. I went there and watched the show with my neighbor. Oprah said, "The Key To Life Is Balance." as a sentence and I just sat there in a moment of WOW. I had just finished my first book named with that same sentence, now coming out of Oprahs mouth. Her saying this was a sign to me that I was on the right track. Of course, I sent my book to Oprah in hopes she would read it and invite me on the show. Unfortunately, I never heard from her. But I loved hearing for the months that followed, "You will be on Oprah!", from friends and clients.

Oprah expressing her inner fears on that show with her weight issues was not only a courageous act but can be looked at as a blessing for us all. No matter how successful we may become, fears of "Am I beautiful?" still come up. I thank her for her honesty and for taking this risk to help each of us see that even in the midst of fear there is opportunity to grow and change. We are all on this path of learning to love ourselves.

Now, this is where I get all "Woo Woo" on you. When connecting with your body, the lower chakras; root, sacral and solar plexus are engaged. These energy centers hold our power, emotional well being, and help in grounding us. When they become out of balance, we cannot love our bellies or our bodies and in turn this affects our spirit; the crown chakra. Being out of balance in your physical body actually means you have been out of balance in your energy field for a longer time. Everything happens in the energy field first. Movement in this area helps to cleanse stagnant and blocked energy which contributes to the holding of these patterns. By gaining control over the abdominal muscles, your core, energetically and physically, will win back your power and you can become confident and fall back in love with yourself. If you want to know more about these energy centers, I have detailed information and an easy guide in The Key To Life Is Balance book.

When starting to connect with the core, it may be difficult to let go of sucking in your belly. As young women, we are taught to look smaller by sucking this part of our bodies. In hiding this precious part of our bodies, we deplete our power in the sacral and solar plexus. Releasing this mind set gives you your power back! When I was in massage school, we were taught that clients with sexual abusive pasts may not want their stomachs massaged. Old emotions of sexual abuse, diet and exercise failures and all your negative thoughts about your body are held there in your core.

Release all of this "old stuff" by connecting with this part of your body. Work out your core and meditate on being ok with it. Let the belly relax as you breathe.

We are all beautiful creations in our own way, here on a journey to give our gifts to others around us and heal ourselves at the same time. Find that beauty inside the core of your being. You do not need to be stuck in these patterns any more.

The most valuable tool you have is the tool of visualization, it is the power of all powers and will help you to take a U turn on your path, when you need it most. This tool is easy and does not cost a penny. All you have to do is to connect with it. Visualization is the most effective and powerful tool I have found. As the law of attraction states, what you focus on, you will receive. Your thoughts will create and form what you are thinking into the physical, because thoughts are energy, and focusing gives the thoughts energy. Giving that thought power and intention, we then manifest what we want to be real. Whether negative or positive, it will show up if you ask for it. So, just be positive so that good things will show up instead of the negative. I am going to reveal three powerful ways I have dealt with my own negative self image.

Using them, you will start to notice changes in your cravings for food and you will find a drive to move your body, whether you dance or exercise.

Changing a pattern like negative body image using visualization, you will want to start at the beginning, where the negativity first began. Think back to your first memory of negative situations that might have triggered a negative body image for you. Using these memories in the following meditation will clear them from blocking your energy and moving it from your body. I like to start with my earliest and work my way forward. At the end of the day, I will look at the situations of the day and work on them so that I am not storing new baggage.

"Insanity: doing the same thing over and over again and expecting different results."
~Albert Einstein

Creating a New Outcome Visualization

Find a comfortable space and sit or lie down, become relaxed, and focus on your breathing.

As you inhale, your belly rises, and as you exhale, it falls. Let go of any holding or sucking in of the belly. See in your mind's eye a situation that brings on a negative self image, feel what pain this memory has in the body. Focus on it as long as you can. Then, take the situation and change it into a positive one. (Example: if someone made a negative comment about your body, change the outcome in your mind to "You are beautiful" instead.) Feel what that feels like, see and feel yourself as beautiful, because you are! You are the only You there is, and You truly are beautiful!

The next one is more than just visualization but is just as easy. It incorporates energy healing. We all have the ability to heal ourselves and others. I have studied Polarity, Reiki and other modalities of this work, each follow the same principal of focusing on unconditional loving thoughts and sending the intention of healing to the one receiving the healing, thus yourself or another.

Loving Gestures Visualization and Healing

Lying in a comfortable and quiet place, focus on your breathing.

Lace your fingers on your belly with the thumbs touching the outside of your navel. Breathing into your belly only loving thoughts, feeling your belly rise and fall with each breath, and being ok with it filling up. Feel like you are letting go of your lower back and feeling the hips becoming light. This helps in balancing energy in your sacral and root Chakras. If you want to ground at this time, think of a root coming from the tail bone, sending it into the Earth.

When you feel the time is right, move your hands to the center of your chest. Place the left hand on the bottom and the right on top. As you breathe, focus on loving energy surrounding your heart center. See this loving energy as white light and see it filling up your heart, creating a huge storage of love inside your chest.

After you are full of love, sit up and wrap your arms around your shoulders. Give yourself a huge hug and say to yourself, "I love you!" When you ready to come back, make sure you have a great attitude about yourself!

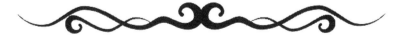

Chapter Eleven
Spa-Cipes for dogs

I have a dog, Jake, and he is a 4 year old rescue dog. A mix of Shar Pei and Chocolate Lab. I have heard Shar peis have dry skin and lots of skin issues as they do not sweat due to their wrinkles. My dog, being half lab, does not have the wrinkles and his skin was itchy and dry and was always biting at his rear, giving him hot spots. I would have to put the cone on him and be after him all the time to stop biting. He created huge sores on his hips, and it was exhausting to deal with.

Then, the calcium bentonite clay came into my life. I was using it on my skin to heal breakouts and drinking it. While learning about the wonderful clay, I started to think that I could use this to heal my dogs problems. I asked around and yes, the clay is safe for dogs to ingest and put on their skin. And yes, it worked! Now my dog gets clay masks, salt scrubs and dog wraps using all of the products I use on myself and my clients.

At first, he was not sure about bath time as it did take a bit longer. When doing the dog wrap, the product needs to sit on the dog up to 15 minutes to work deeply into the fur and skin. But when I am done, my dog jumps and runs! He is so happy, his skin feels good and he smells like he just came from the spa.

Treating dog's skin, instead of giving them a bath, takes a bit more time and the effects last longer. So, it is worth the time it takes. I was having to give him a bath once a week to keep up on his sores, the dry skin flakes and the itching all day long. A regular bath would stop his itching only for a couple of hours. Now, after months and months of treatments, he does not sit on the floor and itch at all. He has not had a breakout hot spot in almost a year.

This chapter is all of the recipes I personally use on my dog Jake. One day, I will add these treatments along with dog massage services to my spa. If you live near my spa and want me to help you with your dog's skin issues, give me a call. I will personally teach you how to heal your dog with my Spa-Cipes for Dogs.

Again, Set N Me Free is a part of my dog's life as well. They have a Pet Wash that is what I use for my Dog wrap. Again, I will list out the active ingredients so you can try to create your own or easily purchase the product itself.

Pet Wash - Aloe barbadensis, Citric acid, Jojoba, Citronella oil

I wet down my dog in the bathtub with warm water and I rub in the pet wash, letting it sit on my dog for up to 15 minutes. I talk to him and tell him to stay so his skin can feel good. Then I rinse him off with warm water.

Use this after a Pet Wash treatment, if the dog has dry skin flakes or has been itching excessively.

Dog Salt Scrub

You will need a bowl and a mixing spoon.
1 cup of Epsom salts
1 cup avocado oil
1 cup olive oil
1 to 3 drops lavender essential oil
1 drop tea tree oil
1 tablespoon vitamin E oil
Rub this entire amount on your dog's fur, rubbing deeply to get down into the skin. He/she will love this part, as it is like scratching his/her back with lots of tiny finger nails. Get all the spots that are dry and flakey. Let the salt and oils sit on your dog up to 5 minutes, then rinse off completely with warm water. Towel him/her dry and then brush in an upward stroke all over the body 3 times. Then in a downward stroke once, and you are done.

Use this clay mask when your dog has hot spots, a growth or lump and/or any skin issue that needs healing. Use on spots where ticks were and on flea bites.

Clay Mask

You will need a bowl, plastic spoon (using plastic when spooning out clay is recommended) and a face paint brush.

1 teaspoon calcium bentonite clay

1 tablespoon aloe or plain water

Mix well until it becomes a paste and cover the skin irritation area. Leave on for as long as the dog will let it sit. If your dog licks it off, it is safe for your dog to ingest. Replace the clay mask two to three times a day until you see the issue clearing up. I put on the mask and I really never wash it off my dog. I let it come off naturally or let him lick it off.

Your dog loves massage! Give him/her some at least once a day to keep muscles and body in a healthy state of being.

If you walk your dog, let your dog run on the beach or open fields, if available. If your dog is left home alone all day, your dog needs massage. Spend at least 15 minutes doing these massage techniques.

Dog Massage

You will need two hands and a willing dog. Have your dog lie on a soft, firm surface such as a rug or mat. You can place a small dog on your lap. Start with several soft, slow strokes from head to tail. When your dog begins to relax, scratch gently behind his ears and move around the face, under the chin, over the nose, between the eyes and over the head. Rub each ear between your thumb and forefinger, too.

Using three fingers, move slowly over the neck, shoulders, and chest in a small, circular motion. With three fingers, softly massage from the buttock to the thigh and down the leg all the way to the paw. Do the front and back of each leg, working your way from top to bottom and then bottom to top.

Place your thumb and index finger on each side of the spine and "walk" toward the base of the tail, and then the outside of each thigh. Finish up with several soft, slow strokes from head to tail.

I give my dog some of what I call Doggie Qigong, and he loves it! Jake is a big dog, about 97 pounds. When he stands in front of me, I start to pat his backside with both of my hands up and down along his spine for a few minutes. Do this several times a day, especially when they get up from a long nap. Qigong helps moves the Chi (energy), this light tapping will help your dog feel great.

Try it on yourself as well or find a Qigong class and learn about this wonderful practice.

As I was writing this book, my dog got skunked and I could not leave you without this important Spa-Cipe! There are old remedies out there that all say they get the odor out. Nothing I have ever used completely takes it away in the moment, the oldest one around being tomato juice, which just sounds like a huge mess to me. I have never tried this one. At the moment I realize my guy has been skunked, I grab the white vinegar bottle and an old cloth. First, you will want to check on your pet to make sure it did not get into their eyes. The skunk's sulfuric spray (mercaptan) will blind your pet for hours and even up to two days. My dog is somewhat schooled on turning his head at the right time and not getting it in the eyes. My cat, on the other hand, once got it so bad he could not open his eyes for four hours.

If your animal gets it in the eyes, you will need to flush the eyes with plain water as much as your animal will allow you to do so. Start with a very wet cloth, blotting the eyes, and then squeezing some water in the corners and drying after each squeeze until you get out as much as you can. Then, place the animal somewhere it will not get hurt while it is blinded, after you give them a complete bath, of course. I always feel so sorry for my animals when they are in this situation. They don't like what you are doing to them, so talk to them, and tell them they are OK. I say things like "You need to stay away from those little striped ones and you know it!" My other cat has never been skunked, I guess he learned. My dog knows better but just cannot resist trying to chase them!

This recipe was created by Paul Krebaum, a chemist and works very well. Sometimes you may have to apply two days in a row to really get the smell out.

Use this when your dog gets skunked.

The Skunk Method

You will need a jar, glass or bowl and an old cloth. Usually you are in a hurry when making this, so grab whatever container you can but it will need to be tall. Sometimes this solution fizzes over.
I will attend to my dogs eyes first, flushing with water if needed. Then I will pour white vinegar on the old cloth and blot the affected area.
1 quart of 3% hydrogen peroxide (I have also used white vinegar)
¼ cup baking soda
1 teaspoon of strong liquid soap such as dishwashing detergent.

Warning
This mixture can be explosive, as it will fizz and creates pressure if it is enclosed in a sealed tight container. Never store unused portion, always discard. Be sure to only mix in an open container and do not try to store or cover it in any way. Do not get the mixture into the dog's eyes, nose or mouth.

After everyone settles down from the excitement and the bath, it will still smell kind of "skunky" in the air. I will take white sage bundles and burn them in the area for up to an hour after. This odor is powerful and will linger for a while. I will also keep lovely smelling candles burning as much as I can all over the house until the smell in the air is gone. Using your natural spray recipes, make one with white vinegar and sage or eucalyptus and spray on any linens your dog may have encountered.

Bonus recipe - Soap Making

I have learned over the years there are many very good soap makers in this area. I am not a soap maker, but I wanted to give you some idea about making your own soap in this book. I asked a client that is a soap maker to give me some of her advice and what follows is what she gave me.

Have fun and *be careful* making your soap!

Mary's Green and Clean Handcrafted Soaps are created with 100% vegetable-based oils and luxuriant butters. The Soap-Maker creates unique recipes enhancing the standard Olive, Coconut and Palm oils with rich butters and oils e.g. Avocado Butter, Avocado Oil, Shea-nut Butter, Cocoa Butter etc... The soaps are crafted to leave skin feeling soft and smooth by utilizing the Cold Process soap-making technique which retains high levels of glycerin and amino fatty acids in the finished product. The soaps are enhanced with both Essential and/or Fragrant oils to add mild fragrances and scents. They are designed to last several weeks when taken care of properly, i.e. in between uses ensure soap bars are stored away from moisture in order to allow the soap to dry.

The Soap Making Process

Caution! Please be sure to **follow all safety guidelines when handling Lye.** If you haven't studied a comprehensive guide on Cold Process soap making, I highly recommend the **Everything Soap Book**. If you are new to cold process soap making, please purchase a book and read about the serious safety issues associated with lye. Another good book to start with is Susan Miller Cavitch's "**The SoapMakers Companion.**"When working with lye, please always use gloves and goggles and do not breathe in the fumes. I also wear long sleeves during my soap making process and keep my goggles on the entire time.

What you will need

- Two large stainless steel pots: one 3 -5 quart and one 16 quart
- One very large stainless steel whisk
- Immersible electric stick blender
- One regular sized stainless steel whisk
- One frothing battery operated whisk
- One hot plate
- 3 - 4 Glass 16 oz measuring cups
- One 8 cup glass measuring cup (for mixing Lye into water. always pour Lye into water never water into Lye)
- One Tare capable scale
- One large hard plastic spatula and a couple of regular sized spatula's
- One candy thermometer (needs to read from zero to 300 degrees)

- 2 15 inch log molds with silicone liners capable of holding 5 pounds of wet soap each (10 lbs) **for**
- **Soap recipe # 1**
- 1 18-Bar-Unfinished-Birchwood-Mold (can be purchased on Brambleberry .com website) **for Soap recipe # 2**
- Log style Soap Cutter or Stainless Steele wire cutter or sharp kitchen knife
- pH strips

Safety equipment
- Safety goggles
- Heavy Duty elbow length rubber gloves
- Long sleeve shirt
- Long pants
- Sturdy boots or shoes and socks
- Dust or Fume resistant mask, for use during Lye into Water mixing, I also use a Facial Shield to protect against lye water, wet soap and soap cleanup splatters.

Work Area:
Needs to be clear of any children and/or pets!
- A minimum of 2 sinks, ideally a double garage work sink is best, you can make soap in a double Kitchen sink but remember that you are working with Lye.
- Two large counter height work areas either 2' by 6' or 2' by 8'

Step by Step Process

1. Setup work area with appropriate utensils stainless steel wire whisks, hard plastic spoons, pots and glass measuring cups, Tare scale and Hot Plate.
2. Fill work sink with Hot water, dish detergent and 2 - 3 cups of white vinegar(lye neutralizer), open window above sink for ventilation.
3. Put on safety attire (see section above).
4. Weigh Distilled Water utilizing 8 cup glass measuring cup on Tare scale and set water into 2nd sink.
5. Weigh Lye utilizing 16 oz glass measuring cup on Tare scale.
6. Slowly pour Lye (Sodium Hydroxide) into water, mixing slowly and thoroughly with regular sized Stainless Steele whisk until water and lye solution starts to clear (3 - 5 minutes), put the empty lye measuring cup into hot water, dish detergent and white vinegar cleaning sink, keep whisk handy as you will further mix the lye water solution until it is clear with no lye particles remaining in the solution.
7. Place Candy Thermometer into Lye / Water solution, initial temperature should be between 150 - 180 degrees Fahrenheit . You want this temperature to come down to around 100 - 105 degrees Fahrenheit.
8. Weigh solid oils in 3 - 5 quart pan utilizing Tare scale, reset for each solid oil being used in the recipe.

9. Place solid oil container on the Hot Plate and set temperature to Medium cover with lid (you will need to check this regularly throughout the process).
10. Monitor regularly both Lye solution and solid oils progress.
11. Place 16 quart Stainless Steel pot on Tare scale. Measure each liquid oil, resetting Tare function for each separate oil. When all liquid oils have been measured, mix thoroughly with large whisk and set aside.
12. Place color oxide, mica etc... into 16 oz measuring cup and pour in 1 -2 tablespoons of carrier oil e.g. Sweet Almond, Sunflower, Olive oil in and mix thoroughly until all of the color powder is dissolved.
13. Once solid oils reach a liquid state, turn off hot plate leaving pot in place.
14. Once lye solution reaches 105 degrees Fahrenheit, pour melted solid oils into large pot of liquid oils and mix thoroughly.
15. Be sure that you have all your safety equipment and soap making attire on.
16. Carefully carry lye solution over to oil pot, and slowly pour lye solution into oils, hand mixing with large whisk, place lye solution glass measuring cup into cleaning sink.
17. Continue to manually mix lye and oils until you see no air bubbles.
18. Place immersible electric stick blender into soap pot completely have setting on medium 4 - 5 and proceed to mix soap mixture, moving blender around the bottom of the soap pot.

19. When soap mixture reaches light Trace (you need to understand Trace stages and have experience in this process stage), using a clean 16 oz. glass measuring cup. Scoop out about 1 cup of wet soap mix and pour into color glass measuring cup, whisk thoroughly until you have a consistent blend of soap mix and color.

20. Check soap pot mixing manually to determine Trace level, if it is still at light trace and you want a solid colored soap bar, add colored soap mixture and mix thoroughly, if you want a swirled affect on the bar the wet soap mix needs to be at medium Trace proceed to pour colored soap mix from high above the pot to low then using large whisk mix from bottom to top lightly (the color will mix more when you pour into the log mold).

21. Pour wet soap mix into log mold evenly into each mold. Using small spatula, contour the top of the soap for an artistic look.

22. Clean all your equipment (keep that safety equipment on!) thoroughly.

23. Most soap batches will process through the saponification within 48 hours and you will be able to un-mold and cut your bars.

Soap Recipe # 1
Lavender Tangerine

Description: Lavender combined with fresh Tangerine fragrance produces a relaxing top note followed up by refreshing middle note scent. The combined oils in this recipe produce a thick and creamy lather.

The following recipe produces nearly 10 pounds of wet soap and requires 2 - 15 inch Log Molds with 5 pound capacity. Any modification or adjustments to this recipe requires a Lye recalculation. You can find Lye calculators on the Web. A good source is the HSCG Web Site:
http://www.soapguild.org/soapmakers/resources/resources.php

Oils
25 oz Coconut Oil Fractionated 76 degree
25 oz Palm Oil
23 oz Olive Oil
23 oz Safflower Oil
6 oz Mango Butter
2 oz Castor Oil

Lye / Water
37.34 oz Distilled Water (this combination is using a 5% Lye discount formulation)
14.77 oz Sodium Hydroxide (**Lye**)

Color
3/4 tsp Apricot Oxide Blush
1 - 2 Tsp of Carrier Oil e.g. Sweet Almond, Grape Seed,
Sunflower etc...

Fragrance
2 Tbsp + 2 tsp Hungarian Lavender Essential Oil
2 Tbsp + 1/2 tsp Tangerine Essential Oil

Molds
2 15 inch log molds with 5 pound capacity

Recipe Tips
1. To create a swirled effect pour color / oil mixture into soap pot at Medium Trace from top to bottom swirling from bottom to top with large wire whisk.
2. Allow bars to set up for 48 hours prior to un-molding.

Soap Recipe # 2
Spa Salt Bar Eucalyptus and Spearmint

Eucalyptus and Spearmint Essential Oils combine to produce a medicinal yet refreshing fragrance. The salts act to pull toxins from the skin as well as act as an exfoliant.

The following recipe produces 12.5 pounds of wet soap and require a 18 bar birch mold with 12.5 pound capacity. Any modifications or adjustments to this recipe requires a Lye recalculation.

Oils
50 oz Coconut Oil Fractionated 76 degree
19 oz Rice Bran Oil
9.5 oz Castor Oil

Lye / Water
28.18 Distilled Water
11.26 Sodium Hydroxide (**Lye**)

Salt
47 oz Calspa Sea Salt
1 cup Pink Himalayan Salt (sprinkled on top for artistic finish)

Color
1 tsp Titanium Oxide

Fragrance
4 Tbs Eucalyptus Spearmint Essential Oil

Molds
1 18 Bar Birch mold with 12.5 pound capacity

Recipe Tips
- Pour wet soap mixture into 18 bar birch mold and then set in the bar separator
- Sprinkle Pink Himalayan salts on each bar for an artistic effect
- Only leave the bars in the mold for 12 hours, as the salt hardens the soap bars very quickly!

Melt and Pour Soap Making

If you are looking for something easy that you can do in your home without much worry about having to deal with Lye, then Melt and Pour Soap Making is for you!

What you will need:
- Melt and Pour white soap base, it can be goats milk or a standard white soap base. I am linking Wholesale Supplies Plus website for reference once there, click on Melt and Pour Soap Base wholesalesuppliesplus.com
- An alternative to the above, you can buy soap base kits where the soap base is already graded and ready to use, this will eliminate the need to grade your soap base.

- A stainless steel double boiler or microwaveable large glass bowl
- A set of stainless steel measuring spoons Tbs - 1/4 Tsp
- 1 large stainless steel whisk
- 1 small 4 oz glass container for holding measured essential oils
- Depending upon the size of your batch 1 - 5 decorative plastic tray molds, you can find these all over the Web. The two vendors I use most often are wholesalesuppliesplus.com or brambleberry.com
- A **Tare** capable scale, where you can reset to zero with an object sitting on it
- Essential oils of choice, this book has many options. I will use Hungarian Lavender and Tangerine in my example. I love these two fragrances together. The combination gives you the calming effects of Lavender combined with the refreshing sweet citrus scent of Tangerine.

Step by Step Melt and Pour Soap Making Process:
1. Measure out essential oils 1 Tbsp + 2 Tsp Hungarian Lavender and 1 Tbsp + 1 Tsp Tangerine into small glass container and mix until well blended. Set aside.
2. If you are using a block of melt and pour base, they usually come in 2 pound blocks. Grade all of your base on a stainless steel cheese grater. If you are using a pre-grated melt and pour, use either the top of your double boiler pot or a large glass bowl to measure out 2 pounds.
3. Place your grated soap base in either your top double boiler pot or a microwave safe glass bowl.

If you are using a double boiler, turn your stove burner to medium and stir until melted into liquid form. If you are using a microwave, place bowl into microwave and set it for 30 second intervals until it is melted.

4. Once the soap is in a melted state, pour in essential oils and whisk until the oils are throughly mixed in. If the melt and pour base starts to solidify, then return it to the microwave or stove top and melt back down.

5. Pour into your molds carefully and scrape off any excess. Repeat with each mold, again if the melt and pour starts to solidify, then return to heat.

6. Let set in molds for 24 hours and pop out of mold. If you are having difficulty releasing the soap from the mold, put the mold in the freezer for about 1/2 hour.

Congratulations! You have complete your first soap project and are ready to use them or give them as gifts!

Bonus Tip : Candle Making

I do have one last tip for you before this book ends.
Candles are expensive and some smell really good but
don't burn all the way. I save all the good smelling
candles that do not finish burning in a bag and then I
get wicks from the craft store. Usually on a rainy or
stormy day, I will pull out my old candle making pans.
Just two old pots I got at the thrift store, and all the
saved candles and my wicks. I will place some water in
the bottom of one of the pans and place the other
inside, making a boiler pot on the stove. I place all of
the jars I have saved in the top pan and turn on the
stove. The smells are amazing when the candles start
to melt. After they melt, pull out old wicks and any
debris. Fill new glass jars or use some of your old ones
with the melted wax. Add in your wick in the middle,
you may have to hold your wick for a minute to keep it
straight. The wax will dry quickly. Voila! You have new
candles and saved money, too.

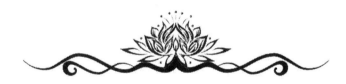

In Closing

I do hope you've enjoyed this book, and the Spa-Cipes in it, along with making sure you given yourself some time and love. Continue to do so.

I have enjoyed writing this book, and I am excited to see more of you giving yourself spa treatments at home.

I have known for about fifteen years that my gift is to relay information in mass form about how to love yourself and have a balanced healthy sense of well being. I strive and succeed at this daily! It does take some dedication, some of your time and most importantly, the willingness, to give them to yourself.

It is all about YOU in this world. Everything you hate and everything you love is all about how you look at the situation. They say there are two sides to the story, meaning everyone sees things differently, depending on their experiences in this life. Whatever it is, it is always a lesson and opportunity to grow and with this growth you will start to love yourself. When you love yourself, you will not allow others to treat you in ways you would not treat yourself.

I have let people treat me poorly in my life time. I learned it and created a pattern of it because I was born into a situation of unhealthy thoughts and boundaries. This created a childhood of low self esteem and kept me stuck in weight issues, depression and more for years. You may have experienced this yourself.

At home spa treatments are the easiest way I have found to pull myself out of that funk, and I do hope you start to use it now that you have more information about treating yourself at home. A perfect time to do a spa treatment is when your mind tells you, "I am bored." This is a great time to give to yourself! Your brain is really just asking for some rejuvenation. I hear people talk about waking up at night and not being able to go back to sleep. A perfect time to make a mask and take a hot bath! I bet it will make you fall asleep as soon as you get out of the tub.

Let this book guide you to learning about yourself. If during one of your at-home spa treatments, negative stuff comes up, or you just cannot turn off the situation that happened to you that day, use my favorite stress reduction meditation. A free download is available on my web site at www.BalanceStudioSpa.com.

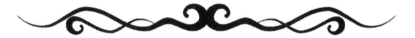

Stress Reduction Meditation

Simply start to picture yourself letting go. Build a box, basket or cabinet in your mind's eye. Place it over your right shoulder. Fill that container with all of your stuff , your stress, your worries. When complete, take in three deep breaths and cut that cord, letting all of your stuff start to float away as you take in more deep breaths.

Bibliography

Balance Studio Spa
BalanceStudioSpa.com
TheKeyToLifeIsBalance.com

Earth's Living Clay
earthslivingclay.com

Set N Me Free
set-n-me-free.com

Cypress Health Institute
cypresshealthinstitute.com

Jan Nelson Design
jannelsonlandscapedesign.com

Theo Jackson - Family Counselor
tjjackson70@netzero.com

Mary's Green and Clean Handcrafted Soaps
squareup.com/market/green-and-clean-soaps

Inara Sophia--CMT, Reiki Master
InaraSophia.com

Dr. Oz: doctoroz.com/videos/better-metabolism-your-body-type

About the Author

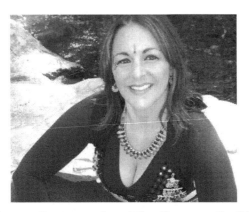

Melissa Stone Santangelo - *The Groovy Goddess,* is the founder of a full service holistic fitness, wellness and skin care center, **Balance Studio Spa**. Located in a serene spot amongst the redwoods of Felton, CA, with flowering gardens and her mosaic art, she created her dream by opening the first of its kind spa in the Santa Cruz Mountains, in 2003.

Certified in Yoga, Pilates, massage and energy work, Melissa is an expert in the field of tender loving care (TLC), detoxification, weight loss and stress reduction. Over the past eleven years, she has led many classes, workshops and written many articles on the subject of holistic care. She wrote a quarterly column in Belly Dance Magazine called Fitness for the Dancer from 2007 until the magazine's end in 2011.

In 2008, she was honored to be asked to produce and co-host a radio show on KSCO 1080AM called Radiance and Chocolate until May 2009. She was able to interview many of her mentors and create a wonderful and powerful show for the community.

At a young age, Melissa knew she would write a book about her journey and she started to journal. In 2008, she self published a book The Key To Life is Balance, a journal of her experiences and more! It shares her journey to enlightenment through finding balance after becoming homeless at 36 with her 5 year old daughter.

Melissa continued to self produce self-help books, videos, and recordings. In 2011, she created The Balance Tool Kit.

In 2013, Melissa created The Balance 7 Day Juice Cleanse meal plan and information about how herbs and food help the body with wellness and balance. This cleanse is inspired by a conversation Melissa had with Jack LaLanne himself. This cleanse can be found in this her second book, Spa-Cipes, The Spa Cookbook. This book includes all of Melissa's holistic recipes to bring her spa to your home.

At the age of 9, Melissa would create spa treatments from food in the kitchen and herbs from the garden when she felt alone and sad. Her teens and early twenties were spent overweight, depressed and lacking in self esteem due to lack of family and community nurturing and support. Becoming homeless was her rock bottom and when she made the decision to go within and make life changes, she came back to her intuition and found a meditation practice that served her. Now, her life long journey is to help others find balance easily and have fun while doing it.

Melissa is a graduate from Cypress Health Institute, class of 2003. She has integrated all of her knowledge with this comprehensive education of massage training and polarity with her Fitness background into a holistic practice she personally uses and teaches.

The Key To Life Is Balance Tool Kit includes:

The Key To Life Is Balance book and work book, Groovy Goddess Yoga and Pilates Workout, Mystic Mediations for Daily Life and Success and Abundance.

BalanceStudioSpa.com

Find Melissa on Facebook at facebook.com/TheGroovyGoddess

Like Balance Studio Spa on Facebook at facebook.com/Balancetoolkit

About the Artist & Editor

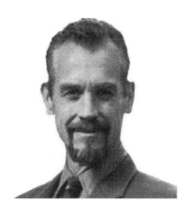

Daniel Gross is a Certified Clinical Hypnotherapist and owner of **Hypnosis Santa Cruz** in Scotts Valley, CA. With a focus on the body's ideal health using the powerful subconscious mind, he has helped hundreds with weight loss, smoking cessation, along with stress and pain reduction. He's created ~HYPNOTIC~ Weight Loss, a one hour seminar and weight loss hypnosis package, and hosts Living Lite Weight Loss Hypnosis seminars throughout the South SF Bay and Santa Cruz areas.

He also loves to create compelling and beautiful things in Photoshop and Word, and is very pleased to have played an integral part in the creation of this book.

To contact Daniel:
daniel@hypnosissantacruz.com
hypnosissantacruz.com
facebook.com/HypnosisSantaCruz

The End

...but only the Beginning

of Your Journey!

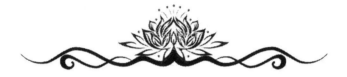

Made in the USA
Charleston, SC
24 June 2014